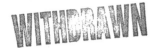

WHAT OTHERS ARE SAYING...

"A comprehensive review of how food allergies affect children's lives, their families, and their school environments. Wonderful tools and resources provided to educate families. A must read for parents of food allergic children!"

—**Dr. Pamela A. Georgeson,**
Allergist with Kenwood Allergy and Asthma Center,
Chesterfield Twp., MI, and media spokesperson for the
American Academy of Asthma, Allergy and Immunology
(AAAAI)

"Food allergies are one of the most serious and complex health issues in America today, especially for children. The more awareness we create among parents, teachers, health professionals and researchers, the more progress we can make to improve the quality of life for food allergic patients."

—**Mike Tringale, MSM, Director of External Affairs,**
Asthma and Allergy Foundation of America
(AAFA)

"For any parent this book provides valuable information about food allergies and their symptoms. It also shows how parents have been able to pursue the issue and get answers about their children's health. This book is a valuable resource for any parent especially with small children. I have also used the information to inform my adult clients who may have had long standing food allergies that they did not identify."

—**Roxanne H. Condon, MS, LPC**
Master of Science, Licensed Professional Counselor

"Thoughtfully written and straight to the point—this is the first book I recommend to parents of children with food allergies. It deals with real world issues not covered in other publications!"

—Deana Boucher, RD CDE, Registered Dietitian and mother of three

"From medical information to personal stories of people living with food allergies...that is what made this book so interesting. Every time I put it down, I couldn't wait to pick it up again to see what I was going to read about next."

—Karen Wolff, LCSW, Licensed Clinical Social Worker and mother of two

"The research is in-depth...writing is clear and concise...grasp of the emotions of parent subjects is intense. Ms. Anderson's writing is hard-hitting at times while similarly gentle and guiding for parents trying their best to protect their children from hidden dangers. You can learn a lot just by reading the sections on the social implications of food-allergic children."

—Maria Duncan, Freelance Writer and mother of two

"Both practical and personal this book is wonderful, giving much needed information and insight to extended family and teachers who care about the 'whole child'."

—Kathleen Reimold, retired teacher and grandmother of four

"I started to tear-up when I was reading—I love the way things are phrased. I am very excited about this book and how it will help parents of children with food allergies."

—Michelle mother of three

THE BOOK THAT STARTED
THE FOOD ALLERGY REVOLUTION

You *can* handle food allergies in your children. You *can* be a successful parent. It *isn't* your fault that your child has food allergies.

Flourishing with Food Allergies provides comfort, guidance and confidence to families more effectively and successfully than any other book. It educates friends, relatives and caretakers of children with food allergies about what is helpful and what is not. The information provided in this book is straightforward and organized to help you.

A. Anderson is the mother of two sons. She is experienced in parenting children with food allergies since both her sons have had them since birth.

Flourishing with Food Allergies is a guide, a reference, and a starting place. It will help you on your unique journey.

FLOURISHING WITH FOOD ALLERGIES

SOCIAL, EMOTIONAL,
AND PRACTICAL GUIDANCE FOR
FAMILIES WITH YOUNG CHILDREN

A. ANDERSON

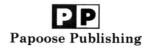

Papoose Publishing

Copyright © 2008 by A. Anderson

All rights reserved.

Printed in the United States of America

No part of this book may be reproduced or transmitted in any form or by any means, electronic or mechanical, including photocopying, recording or by any information storage and retrieval system, without written permission from the author, except for the inclusion of brief quotations in a review. For information about permission to reproduce selections from this book write to Permissions, Papoose Publishing 385 Main Street South, Suite 404-200, Southbury, CT 06488.

For orders see www.flourishingwithfoodallergies.com

ISBN 978-0-615-18704-4

This book is intended to present the research and ideas of its author. If a reader requires personal advice, he or she should consult a competent professional. The author and publisher disclaim liability for any adverse effects resulting directly or indirectly from information contained in this book.

Library of Congress Cataloging-in-Publication Data

Anderson, A.
Flourishing with Food Allergies: Social, Emotional and Practical Guidance for Families with Young Children.
Includes bibliographical references.
ISBN 978-0-615-18704-4 (trade paperback)

2008921118

TABLE OF CONTENTS

FOREWORD

This book is useful for parents, grandparents, aunts, uncles, friends, teachers, caretakers, doctors, chefs and anyone in a service industry who comes into contact with children such as those in schools, restaurants, resorts and travel.

There are probably children who you see everyday who suffer from food allergies, but you wouldn't know it. It is not something that is spoken of out of the blue, unless there is a reason to do so. This book will enhance your understanding of how it feels to have a child with a food allergy as well as the practical aspects of eating at friends' and relatives' houses, restaurants and schools. The guidance provided can help you to become a better parent, relative, friend, teacher or service provider.

We brought two children into the world during the past five years. I never imagined or knew of the love that I would feel for our sons. I never expected that our sons would have food allergies and that I would feel alone and a bit lost at times. While I have found various aspects of parenthood to be challenging, dealing with our sons' food allergies is perhaps one of the most challenging. It causes me to question myself, others and really think about risks. Despite the worries, I feel overwhelmingly blessed to have two adorable sons and a great partner for a husband.

If you know and care about a child who has a food allergy, then you can learn how to help that child and family by obtaining a better understanding of what it is like to care for and love a child with food allergies. I detail the journey my husband and I took on with our two sons. I also include many interviews with other parents of children with food allergies which may help you identify similar symptoms and situations. These interviews share the shock parents had while learning that their child has an allergy as well as successes in how they handle their situations. Each family handles their child's food allergies differently and with varying caution, confidence and optimism. Some are very careful while others take more risks and are willing to deal with an allergic reaction. Additionally, I extensively researched food allergies on interesting topics related to the "Big Eight" of dairy, egg, peanut, tree nut, soy, wheat, fish and shellfish.

If your child or children have food allergies, then this book can provide you with a sense of friendship in a world undergoing a food allergy crisis or even an epidemic. Knowing that you are not alone is often a great comfort. I hope that by sharing my family's experiences and other parents' experiences that yours can be improved. This book provides social, emotional and practical guidance to everyday situations and feelings.

PREFACE

If a child in your life has been diagnosed with food allergies, you may feel worried, alone and confused about the seriousness of the allergy. As parents, we only want what is best for our children. Sometimes people suggest actions which don't agree with our maternal or paternal instinct. I believe this book can bring you a sense of comfort and can relieve some of your anxieties as you decide what is best for you and your child by reading about experiences of parents who have raised a child with food allergies.

When I learned of our sons' food allergies, I felt alone and anxious. I searched for books that would help me deal with this situation, but the only books I found were medical books or recipe books. Some of the descriptions were frightening and immediately turned me off. I wanted to be empowered to handle our sons' food allergies with confidence. Therefore, I wrote this book with the goal of providing social, emotional and practical guidance to empower parents and caretakers of food allergic children.

Emotional guidance is provided through mothers sharing their stories of how the discovery of food allergies emerged. These stories include details of a child's reactions to foods as well as how the parents and doctors handled the child's reactions. Their stories and successes will help you by demonstrating that children with food allergies can and do flourish. Additional emotional guidance is provided through an interview with a psychotherapist, as well as interviews with four medical doctors, each providing positive statements about handling food allergies from the child's and parents' perspectives. A chapter especially for dads, written by my husband, from a father's point-of-view is included as well.

Social guidance is provided by exploring ideas for social situations such as birthday parties, school and play dates in which food is involved. Ideas for food-free toddler activities are suggested as well. The question of whether a parent can find a safe preschool environment is explored as is the option for home-schooling your preschooler. Once a food allergic child enters kindergarten, the options for preparing various action plans and communicating with the teacher are explained.

Practical guidance is provided by explaining how food allergens and ingredients can be identified so that those foods can be carefully avoided at the grocery store. The book also offers information about airline travel guidelines and recommendations for preparing for travel and keeping your child safe. Ideas are explored about the various possible affects of food allergies such as ADHD, autism and asthma. Further questions surrounding pesticides, antibiotics, hormones and genetically modified foods that might lead to the increased incidence of food allergies in our children are explored as well.

The final goal of this book is to bring a heightened level of awareness in the United States to food allergies. We need to ask our government to allocate funding for more research. There is a sample letter in the conclusion of the book that you may copy and send to your congressman or woman to ask that he or she represent your concerns about food allergies to our federal government.

ACKNOWLEDGEMENTS

I sincerely thank all of the fine parents who shared their stories, successes, feelings and frustrations for the interviews in this book. Many thanks to Karen, Jennifer, Larissa, Heather, Kathy, Yael, Ornit, Cassie, Stephanie, Diane, Michelle, Catherine, Michelle, Katie, Rachelle and Ria. I know each hopes her story will help others.

I am grateful for the professionals, Dr. Schultz, Dr. Burton, Dr. Alder, Dr. Kwittken, Dr. Berry, Tricia Dannenhoffer and Angela Racine who provided their expertise and experience through the interview process. The doctors, therapist and teachers provide valuable perspectives.

Special thanks go to Nancy Manning who edited this book ease and speed—a true gift. Additional thanks go to Maria Duncan for suggesting that I write about food allergies, Jeany Mui for her ideas and Kathy Reimold for proofreading the book. Many thanks to Foltz Design for their generous time and book cover.

Finally and most importantly, many thanks to my husband for sharing his written perspective, proofreading, web skills and providing support with all of the details. Thanks to my beautiful and amazing sons who inspired me to write this book.

WARNING—DISCLAIMER

The contents of this book are not intended to provide medical advice. Medical advice should be obtained from a qualified health professional. No treatment action should be undertaken without consultation with a physician. Each patient is different. These testimonies are just some of my and others' collective experiences or clinical knowledge.

The author of this book is not a doctor or medical professional. The author has no medical training. The author is a mother who is sharing her experiences and the experiences of other non-medical mothers and fathers. The author and contributors to *Flourishing with Food Allergies* do not assume any liability for the contents of material provided. Reliance on any information provided by this book is solely at your own risk. We assume no liability or responsibility for damage or injury to persons or property arising from any use of any product, information, idea, or guidance contained in the materials provided to you.

In no way should *Flourishing with Food Allergies* be considered as offering medical advice. No one should disregard medical advice or delay in seeking it because of something you have read in this book. It should not be used in place of a call to, consultation with, advice from or visit with your physician or other qualified health care provider. This book does not specifically recommend or endorse any test, products or procedures that have been mentioned. Some information may be out of date. The information should not be considered complete, nor should it be relied on to suggest a course of treatment for a particular individual.

Flourishing with Food Allergies does not provide medical advice on the history, causes or treatment of food allergies. It provides social, emotional and practical guidance for parents and caretakers of food allergic children. The information and experiences expressed in this book are general in nature and are provided for informational purposes only. Please consult your own physician or appropriate health care provider

INTRODUCTION

No one is sure why food allergies are on the rise in the United States, especially for our children. But food allergies are indeed on the rise. "The prevalence of peanut allergies has doubled in the five years from 1997 to 2002 according to research reported in the...Journal of Allergy and Clinical Immunology and researchers don't really know why."[1] Research is ongoing to determine the cause for the increase of food allergies. According to the Food Allergy and Anaphylaxis Network, scientists believe that less than *one* percent of the population was affected by a food allergy ten years ago.[2] Today, the number of people with food allergies is *four* percent or 11.4 million Americans,[3] which falls between cancer and diabetes rates in the chart below.

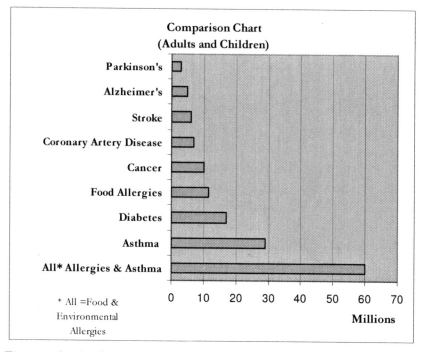

Figures obtained from FAAN, FDA and AAFA.[4]

In the United States, food allergy rates are higher in children than in adults. According to the National Institutes of Allergy and Infectious Diseases, six to eight percent of school aged children have food allergies.[5] According to the Asthma and Allergy Foundation of America eight percent of preschool aged children have food allergies.[6] Why? One study found that children born of women over the age of twenty-nine are about three times more likely to have food allergies, according to the Children's Hospital Boston's Allergy/Immunology program between 1998 and 2000.[7] A history of family allergies will increase the likelihood that offspring will have allergies.

Food allergies are different from food intolerances: They are more serious and can result in anaphylactic shock. A food allergy exists when the immune system kicks into action as a "defense" to the food and creates an IgE antibody to attack the food in the blood stream. Ninety percent of food allergies are caused by eight foods: Dairy, soy, eggs, wheat, peanuts, tree nuts, fish and shellfish. The most severe reactions occur with peanuts and tree nuts, according to Massachusetts Department of Education. U.S. emergency rooms handle roughly 30,000 allergic reactions each year. Our families suffer from over 150 deaths each year.[8]

Food allergies, especially in our youngest members of society, are becoming an epidemic. This epidemic is silently growing. Disbelief among parents, grandparents and much of society fuels the epidemic as we watch it happen. We, as a society, need to embrace this invisible disability. We need to support each other socially and emotionally while the medical and scientific answers are being found. We also need to ask whether food allergies can manifest in disorders such as autism, ADHD and asthma. We need to ask our government to allocate more funding for programs on food allergies and then encourage our medical community to research why food allergies are on the rise.

A positive step is that the United States Government improved labeling laws to help us identify allergens in foods. Laws have been put into place by the USDA, which state that as of January 1, 2006, the

Food Allergen Labeling and Consumer Protection Act of 2004 (FALCPA) became effective. The law required manufacturers to identify clearly on their food labels if a food product has any ingredients that contain protein derived from any of the eight major allergy foods and food groups: Dairy, soy, eggs, wheat, peanuts, tree nuts, fish and shellfish.[9] But we should still be wary of catch-all ingredients, "Any natural flavor is normally quite complex, with dozens or hundreds of chemicals interacting to create the taste/smell."[10] Can you imagine eating a food with three hundred ingredients? How can we be sure that some of these ingredients aren't derived from a food allergen? Who is performing quality control on all of these ingredients?

Also consider the effect of genetically modified foods, pesticides, chemicals, antibodies and hormones that are put into our foods and ultimately our own bodies. What we put into our bodies can make all the difference in the world. A body's reaction to food is a mystery that needs to be solved, especially for our most precious children.

When children have reactions, most parents interviewed for this book were frustrated with the conflicting viewpoints of doctors and test results. For instance, when my son was blood tested for a dairy allergy, the result was negative. But when he was skin prick tested a week later, the result was positive. Numerous other parents have experienced similar confusion when doctors have recommended ultimately unnecessary x-rays, intestinal biopsies and seizure tests. Doctors and parents need a reliable way to determine if a child has food allergies rather than guessing. Healthcare costs could be reduced for everyone if unnecessary, expensive and sometimes dangerous tests could be avoided. We need an accurate non-invasive test that won't trigger a food allergy in an infant or young child.

We need to ask and show our support for food allergy research. On May 12, 2008, Anthony S. Fauci, M.D., Director of the National Institute of Allergy and Infectious Diseases at the National Institutes of Health, states in an article entitled, *Raising Awareness of the Personal and Re-*

search Challenges of Food Allergy, "Much progress has been made in the scientific understanding of food allergies and in the public's awareness of how to manage them. But for millions of individuals, especially children, food allergies continue to limit their activities and threaten their health and lives. As we observe Food Allergy Awareness Week, we need to *redouble* our efforts to understand food allergies and reduce the limitations and suffering they impose on people who have them." Then, on May 14, 2008, Dr. Fauci gave testimony at the U.S. Senate hearing for the Subcommittee on Children and Families Committee on Health, Education, Labor, and Pensions, where he estimated $13.4 million might be spent on food allergy research in 2008 and explained the seriousness of the problem and need for more funding.[11]

Two years ago, we were in a similar state of need. In June 2006, it was reported by The Chicago Tribune, "Dr. Scott Sicherer, of Mt. Sinai School of Medicine in New York City stated, 'There are no studies looking in this country at whether the rate of food allergies has increased over long periods of time.' The National Institute of Allergy and Infectious Diseases, part of the National Institutes of Health, announced last year it would spend *$17 million over five years* for a food allergy research consortium at Mt. Sinai in New York. Spending on food allergy research by the allergy institute more than doubled last year to $7.7 million. But that remains a paltry sum, according to the researchers who gathered at Children's Memorial on Wednesday, *who called on Congress to allocate $50 million annually* for food allergy research. 'There are enough children with food allergies to do the thorough research needed to determine not only how many are now affected, but also to find better treatments,' said Dr. Robert Schleimer, chief of the Allergy-Immunology Division at Northwestern University Feinberg School of Medicine."[12]

Six years ago, in 2002 according to the Pew Initiative on Food and Biotechnology's conclusions and recommendations, "While several federal agencies contribute independently to food allergy research, it does not appear to be a priority for any of them. There were only thirty-three research projects supported by the federal government at the time this analysis was conducted, with a total research effort in the range of $4.2 to $7 million. This is a limited commitment in relation to both the research needs on this topic and to the total federal commitment to biomedical and related life science research in fiscal year 2001 of $18.2 billion (AAAS 2001)."[13]

In contrast, it appears the most impressive research that has been widely organized is the EuroPrevall study of food allergies, which accepted the following participating countries: Italy, Switzerland, Iceland, Ghana, Germany, Lithuania, Spain, Austria, Sweden, Bulgaria, the Netherlands, United Kingdom, Denmark, Poland, Greece, France, New Zealand, Australia, Russia, India and China. In June 2005, the work of the E.U. (European Union) Integrated Project EuroPrevall was started. EuroPrevall is the largest research project on food allergy ever performed in Europe. Major aims of this project are to generate for the first time reliable data on the prevalence of food allergies across Europe and on the natural course of food allergy development in infants.[14] Although it is not the intention of EuroPrevall to expand to the United States, we can ask our government to initiate major research on food allergies.

In the United States, there are several organizations whose focus is food allergies such as the Food Allergy and Anaphylaxis Network (FAAN), Asthma and Allergy Foundation of America (AAFA), American Academy of Allergy Asthma and Immunology (AAAAI), and Food Allergy Initiative (FAI). You can help these organizations and The National Institute of Allergy and Infectious Diseases by supporting their requests for more funding when you write to your congressmen and congresswomen to request more funding for food allergy research. In the conclusion there is a sample letter you may use for this purpose.

PART 1: THE PROBLEM

Our Story

INTRODUCTION

Last night I had a dream, or perhaps a nightmare, that my mother, whom I love very much, was babysitting my two young sons, and she gave them some candies. There was candy such as banana flavored taffy, lollipops, sweet tarts and all sorts of things that I had never seen before. My children were grabbing the candy and gleefully eating it. In my dream, I ran around the room screaming at my mother that I did not know what was in this candy and she had no right to give it to them without checking with me first. She nonchalantly responded that the boys would be fine. She shrugged, frowned a little bit, like I was a bit crazy, and casually tried to calm my fears by saying, "Oh, don't worry."

I woke up in a sweat. Adrenaline was surging through my arms and legs, giving my fingers a tingly sensation. I tried to remind myself that this was only a dream. I then tried to relax and go back to sleep, but it was impossible. I was wired, nervous and awake for the duration of the night. This dream summed up the main fear that I have, that the people I trust most might not fully understand the severity of an allergy. They might accidentally put my children's lives at risk. They might interpret my husband's and my behavior as over-reactive, over-protective and just basically a bit crazy.

At times that nightmare seems like reality as I face another day. Other times, it really isn't that bad. Keeping things in perspective and keeping a positive attitude have helped my husband and me the most in dealing with both of our sons' food allergies. Both of our boys have a dairy, egg and chicken allergy. We've also been advised to avoid peanuts and tree nuts hopefully to fend off an allergy if we wait until the children are school-aged before introducing these potentially serious allergens.

We have found that dairy is our most difficult challenge. Not only was our first son's reaction to dairy serious, but we found that dairy is in almost everything we eat in our popular culture. It is disguised under names such as casein, whey and lactic acid, just to name a few. These items are used in what seems like all prepackaged foods including crackers, cereals, cookies, cakes, and breads. Furthermore, we never realized what a dairy-oriented society we live in with popular treats as pizza, ice cream, cheeseburgers and nacho-cheese snacks prevalent at most parties.

For awhile, I did not want to write about these allergies or my experiences with them. It was too painful and emotionally exhausting for me. I felt that the last thing I wanted to do during my "down" time when the children were napping or asleep for the night was to sit down with my word processor and re-live the fears and frustrations of the day with respect to their allergies.

I am glad that I waited. Now that my sons are a little older and I am not so tired from just having had babies, I have the energy to take a deep breath and sit down at the keyboard and feel positive. My sons are two and four as of this writing. We have been entrenched in dealing with these allergies for more than three years. Now, I feel I am ready to share my story and my feelings.

This is not a story of how hard or terrible things have been. Rather, it is a story of a mother and father who were forced to go on a path they had never imagined. So many surprises exist with parenthood. Before having children, we had no idea how much we would love them and often we stare at them in awe and happiness. We had never thought of having to deal with food allergies. We learned the name for these food allergies is the "invisible disability." It is an accurate name because it is something that affects the child's ability to function normally in our society, but no one can see the problem from just looking at the child, unless, of course, he or she sees the child having a reaction to the food. In spite of the food allergies, our sons are flourishing. They are healthy, bright, happy and loving children.

This experience has opened our eyes to our own diet and food reactions, as well as improved our own health. We have learned how to change our own diets to support our children's food allergies. This experience has also taught us about other people's attitudes, ignorance and compassion or lack thereof. We have found wonderful and supportive friends and members of our families. Our story is about feeling empowered to handle our children's food allergies in a world that is filled with foods seemingly benign, but dangerous to our most beloved.

CHAPTER 1: BEFORE BABIES

One morning, while at work, I was in the office kitchen getting a cup of coffee. A friend of mine walked in and was wearing a new black leather jacket. "What a great jacket," I told him. He said he picked it up in Europe, where he just had traveled with his friend. "You should go to Europe—you'd love it," he said to me. As I walked back to my desk, I thought, "I should!" I sat down and sent a one-line email to my sister that read, "Wanna go to Paris?" Within a few minutes, she replied, "Okay!"

So we were off, making plans, selecting a date. We decided to go soon, after taxes were due and during the nice weather in May—just after my husband's birthday. During those next four weeks, my husband's father passed away from a heart attack after suffering from Parkinson's disease for over ten years. The temperature grew to ninety degrees while my husband and his siblings planned their father's funeral. About five years earlier, we had moved across the country to be closer to my husband's father to support him during his last years of life. We were both so glad that we had been around to help him plant a garden each summer, mow his lawn and bring dinner over once in a while from his favorite restaurants.

My husband and I had been married for ten years, after having dated for five years. During those fifteen years, we went to school together during the evening hours to earn some graduate certificates in the fields of law and information technology. We worked as paralegals, and then moved into the computer field, just as the Internet was emerging. My husband started a computer consulting business, and I joined him in this exciting and challenging adventure. Eventually, we sold our successful business and took jobs at a large computer company so that we could move closer to both of our families. I knew that I wanted to have children and that once we did, moving would be difficult.

Now, my sister and I were to fly to Paris for a long dreamed of trip to the exciting city. Paris was great—we learned how to take the subway and zipped all over the city. My favorite site was the Palace of Versailles. The Hall of Mirrors at the Palace was lined with huge mirrors and chandeliers that reflected the gorgeous gardens below. The food was fabulous in Paris as well. My sister and I were sure to eat a good breakfast everyday, then I was always eager for lunch and dinner too. I especially remember the steak dinner the first night, the eggs for breakfast with fresh greens and French bread as well as the egg rolls and other snacks we nibbled on along the way.

As the week went on, I began to suspect that I might be pregnant. I called my husband and mentioned my suspicion to him. Still reeling from the shock of his father's death, I felt that he wasn't too sure what to think. When I returned home, I found out, for sure, that I was pregnant—and I was thrilled. When I told my husband the news, we kissed and neither of us really knew what to expect.

For the next nine months, I ate and ate—fruits, vegetables, meats, cheese, peanut butter, ice cream, milk, yogurt and just about anything that I wanted. I tried to eat high quality foods such as salmon and good cuts of beef. I avoided fast food restaurants and only ate there out of desperate hunger once or twice when too far from home. I loved eating berries, as it was summer time when I was starting my pregnancy. I gained about forty pounds during the nine months and did not experience much morning sickness. But I was exhausted most of the time, and my muscles ached terribly with even the slightest exercise or strain. My doctor assured me that all was well and my weight gain and girth growth were normal. Finally, one week before my due date on a cold January day, I went into labor.

I was at home for the first twenty-four hours of labor, then my water broke and I went to the hospital around midnight. It was freezing outside, but the hospital was warm and friendly. The emergency room receptionist was expecting me as I came through the door and actually greeted me by name and with a smile. I love small towns. The labor during the night was long and painful. The nurse stayed by my bedside all night long monitoring the contractions and making sure that the baby and I were fine. She was sweet and supportive. I was given Demerol, and later an epidural, which did not really work, since I could still fully feel the contractions and my legs quite clearly.

Finally at about two o'clock the following afternoon, after thirty-six hours of labor, I gave birth to our amazing son who weighed seven pounds nine and one-half ounces and cried vibrantly. He was so beautiful. His eyes were slanted and opened and closed so wonderfully, I could hardly believe that he was mine. I was so lucky and proud to be his mother. I breastfed him from the start and asked that they wake me up during the night so that I could feed him, which they did.

CHAPTER 2: OUR FIRST SON

My new son's pediatrician advised me not to eat tomatoes, dairy and chocolate as these foods had a tendency to make a baby gassy and irritable. I asked the doctor how far away to stay from these foods. He replied, "Completely." I said, "Even a piece of cheese on a sandwich is no good?" He assured me that even a piece of cheese on a sandwich was to be avoided. I guessed that I needn't ask about the pizza that I'd been having every Friday night for the past fifteen years with my husband. This advice was a bit alarming to me and I didn't like the idea of having to modify my diet. I followed his advice, but only to a certain extent. I would cheat here and there.

I must admit that in retrospect, this advice was excellent. But, I only moderately followed his advice. I am sure I ate cheese on a few sandwiches, butter on my broccoli, and ice cream in front of the television while laughing at the show "Sex and the City." While I considered myself to be a healthy eater because I did not drink soft drinks or eat a lot of junk food or fast food, I could have done better. I did not believe that my diet should be changed so drastically, nor did I want to change it. I was happy with the foods that I liked and felt that I was generally in good health.

Our son gained several pounds the first month and the second month. By the third month he had only gained one pound. During this month I had also begun to try to get him on a schedule of feeding to promote a better sleeping schedule. I had read that if the child can eat more at one time, then there will be more time between feedings, which will allow him to sleep longer during the night. (I was tired.)

In pursuing this goal, I began to use a pacifier and would stretch out his feeding time an extra twenty minutes or so from the time he began to fuss during the day. At night, I would feed him immediately. Eventually, his feeding time would move closer to every two or three hours, as was my goal. Although a schedule was beginning to develop, I was entirely disappointed during the doctor's appointment; my precious baby had gained only one pound that third month. I felt that I had failed. I had worked so hard that month to pay extra attention to his feeding and sleeping, but felt I might have hurt him instead. Perhaps I had not fed him enough. I did not know.

I discovered a similar situation in my family history. My cousin was placed in the hospital as an infant for lack of weight gain around the third month. He would vomit after drinking milk and eventually required hospitalization. My aunt switched him from cow's milk to soy milk and was successful in nursing him back to health. My cousin was not breastfed, but probably did receive some dairy during the pregnancy. My aunt advised me that both my cousin and his father were allergic to dairy and eggs as babies. As an adult, my aunt believes her son remains lactose intolerant and he avoids dairy products. My uncle recalls, "I was hospitalized once as an adult when I ate some Tile fish along with two martinis. I don't know if it was anaphylactic shock, but I had trouble breathing."

So perhaps my son's lack of weight gain during his third month wasn't due to my implementing a feeding schedule. Instead it may have been in his genes and our family history. Was the cause of my son's food allergy genetic? Was the allergy made worse because I did not heed the advice of my son's pediatrician strictly enough? Perhaps it was a combination of the two.

I highly recommend asking relatives about food allergy history. For some reason, it took me several years to learn about these allergies. I should have asked my family members earlier and made the phone calls sooner. Although my grandmother was no longer alive to fill in the details of my uncle's allergy, my aunt was able to provide the information about him and my cousin.

Our son had some difficulty eating right from the start. Often he would cry and I would try to feed him, but he seemed uninterested. After more crying, I would try something else, like changing his diaper or holding him in a different way. My husband would throw out suggestions, such as, "Why don't you try feeding him again?" Sometimes I would feel frustrated from confusion, since I had just tried to feed him not five minutes earlier, and now I was to try again? So I would protest saying, "I just tried that!" shouting above the crying. But then I'd try again and nine times out of ten he would eat eagerly after several attempts.

In retrospect, I wonder if our son suffered from cramps and gas. Perhaps he was hungry but at the same time was wary of eating. Perhaps the breast milk had some dairy in it that made him gassy. I wouldn't say that he was colicky because his crying did not last for hours, but when he cried he really let loose. Further, his crying did not cease after the first three months, but continued for years when he was over-tired or over-hungry.

In addition to some strong bouts of crying, our son had eczema. He developed a red bumpy rash on his legs and arms. The pediatrician gave us some prescription strength non-steroid cream, which helped to clear it up. We would slather him with a thick off-the-shelf cream also recommended, to prevent the rash from reappearing. I am not sure if this rash was caused by food allergies, dry skin, soap residue or dryer fabric sheet residue, all of which our doctor postulated.

His eczema worsened during the winter months. I believe he was sensitive to detergents and fabric softeners. We were advised not to use fabric softener sheets in the dryer because they leave a film on the clothing. So after washing all the clothing before he was born, I had to re-wash everything not too long after he was born. Interestingly, I received a funny email about the various uses of dryer fabric softeners, above and beyond softening clothing. For instance, softeners could be used to ward of bugs by rubbing them on your skin or hanging them in a tent while camping. There were a variety of other odd uses. Obviously, fabric softener drier sheets are toxic. Even bugs want nothing to do with them.

We now use the liquid fabric softener in the rinse phase of the washing machine. I am also careful to use the "free of scents" variety to avoid perfumes or other irritants.

Another mistake I made was to believe that all of the special and expensive baby products were good for my baby. We were bombarded with so many samples of baby shampoos, baby washes, lotions, cleansers, diaper creams and powders, that it was truly perplexing. Most of these products were perfumed and had different colors. My mother and the doctor would chuckle at my confusion saying that when they were young parents, they did not have so many choices so it really wasn't an issue.

Another contributing factor to the eczema might have been the pink bottled bubble bath we thought was fun to use in our son's bathtub once he was about a year old. Again, the doctors said to eliminate all soaps and bubble baths that contained dyes and perfumes. He recommended the same gentle liquid cleanser that my dermatologist had recommended. That was enough proof for me to switch both of us to this cleanser. Our doctor also suggested that we rinse our son with clean water from the tub tap before removing him from the bath to get any residue from soap or shampoo off of him.

My advice to new mothers is not to use expensive brands with pretty packaging and colors, but rather just to use a very small quantity of a tearless shampoo and a non-irritating cleanser for the body that has the least number of ingredients, dyes and perfumes. Certainly the baby can't tell what color the shampoo is and probably can't even smell it. The packaging is probably for the mother. A baby can be cleaned with water and a touch of simple soap. Just a gentle washcloth with water in a tub does a great job.

While soap residue, dryer fabric sheets and dry skin might have made his eczema worse, I believe the true cause of the skin condition was the allergic reactions he was experiencing from the breast milk that contained foods to which he later tested positive. My layperson's understanding is that eczema is an allergic symptom. It is caused by the inability of the infant's immature digestive system to digest certain proteins, such as the dairy proteins, which can be hard to break down. These hard-to-digest proteins travel through the digestive system and go into the blood stream undigested. The liver then tries to cleanse the blood stream of this undigested protein. This works for a while, but then the liver becomes overloaded and cannot clean the bloodstream sufficiently. As a result, the immune system comes to the rescue and builds antibodies to attack the foreign proteins. Once the immune system creates antibodies, the allergic reaction is in place. The immune system's antibodies tell the body to attack that foreign substance as if it were a virus or disease, which can cause the infant's body to go into overdrive, possibly resulting in anaphylactic shock. In the meantime, this foreign substance still needs to be excreted from the infant's body, so the skin is used for excretion rather then the digestive system. Thus the skin becomes the cleanser of the body and shows a rash as the foreign substance comes out.

While our son's eating, sleeping and eczema improved over several months, I tried to adjust from full time professional to full time stay-at-home mother. It was perplexing at times. While I loved to feed, hold, photograph and kiss my beautiful baby, I also became a bit lonesome for adult interaction, getting out of the house everyday, and the short term accomplishments to which I'd grown accustomed after having worked for fifteen years. In my mind and my heart, I now had everything I'd been working for over the past ten years, but it was difficult to change the get-up-and-go rhythm to which my body and mind had grown accustomed. Furthermore, my desire to achieve and accomplish was no longer being met in the same way. Now I was focusing on a larger, longer range goal instead of meeting milestones on a project plan.

During the first two months I did not get out much at all because it was cold and I was wary of bringing our son to places where he might get sick. I busied myself with reading books on infant sleep and feeding habits. Then I joined a mother's group at the end of two months. After three months, to help my mental and physical state, I joined a health club with childcare. I had my sights set on returning to work at seven months. This plan was discussed and jointly agreed upon by my manager prior to my leaving work. My manager and I were happy with this plan and I loved my job so had every intention of returning. Furthermore, my husband and I had just purchased a home two years earlier, so we needed my salary. So, in accordance with the plan, I began to evaluate the childcare centers in the area when our son was about eight weeks old.

Chapter 3: The Discovery

Making the decision to return to work was most difficult. I considered not returning but felt I'd be throwing away fifteen years of hard work and another five to six of education. Discovering that our child had food allergies played a role in the decision. But I am confident that our decision would have been right for us and him even if he had no food allergies.

I began to research daycare centers in the area. I selected three or four to visit and began my search on a cold, snowy day in March. There was a traffic jam for several miles and I was stuck for about one-half hour to go just a short distance. I called the daycare center from my car. The administrator was kind and suggested that I turn around and come to visit another day instead. But I insisted that I was still coming. True to my word, however foolish, I finally arrived. When I was being shown around, I saw the children in their rooms with their daycare providers. The little faces would turn quickly to see who was coming, only more slowly to turn back in a quiet, disappointed way. It really broke my heart. I felt that each child longed for his or her mother to be walking through that door and was so disappointed to see yet another stranger.

Despite my doubts, I persisted in visiting the other daycare centers and eventually narrowed the choice down to two centers that seemed to be in a good locale, with decent providers and at a moderate cost. I wanted my husband involved so we made another visit to both these centers together. Once there, we stood holding our son's infant car seat, while he slept. We felt confused and perplexed at these environments. The people seemed so nice and the children seemed somewhat happy or at least entertained. But our hearts ached as we tried to make a decision. I was constantly disappointed at how small a seven-month-old child was because I hoped he would be more self-sufficient, walking, and talking. I had no idea how long it takes for children to grow up. I would ask the providers, "How old is that one, and this one?" The thought of leaving my son at that size just did not settle well with me. I was terribly confused as to what the right thing was to do. I asked a new mommy friend of mine how she felt after returning to her airline pilot career. She replied, "Sometimes the break is nice, but sometimes I miss my son, too." I wanted a definitive answer, but found none.

Our son was about four or five months old when I decided to start weaning him so that I could return to work. He had not yet tried drinking from a bottle. I decided to give him some formula since we had several cans of it in our cupboard from free promotional gifts handed out at the birthing classes at the hospital. I read the instructions, mixed the formula and put it in a bottle. I held my son and let him chew on the bottle's nipple a bit. He took a bit here and there, never more than one or two ounces at a time. This went on for perhaps a week or two, until my son flat out refused to be given the bottle and decided that it was a hateful thing. He screamed bloody murder if I tried to give it to him. Sometime the screaming fits would last for twenty minutes, probably just until he was sure I knew how mad he was. Then the only thing that would bring him any peace was to breastfeed him immediately.

I concluded at that time that indeed my son was "not of a mild temperament" as described by our pediatrician on one early visit. I became apprehensive about giving him a bottle and having to deal with twenty minutes of crying. Sometimes just seeing the bottle would set him off. After several weeks of these unsuccessful attempts, I tried a different tack. Instead of holding him, I placed him in his little vibrating rocking chair and tried to give him the bottle while sitting in front of him.

He seemed to like this technique a little better. He chewed and sucked on the bottle's nipple for several minutes. I noticed that his shirt became a bit wet around the neckline from all the dribbling and drooling and he'd start to cry a bit, so I brought him up to the bathtub afterward for a clean up. As I bathed him, I noticed that his neck was red and the skin slightly raised. I worried that the bath water was too warm or that he had worked himself up from crying. I did not know why his neck would be red. The color vanished within a few minutes, so I relaxed.

I prepared his formula and gave him the bottle the next evening. His shirt neckline became wet from the drool and dribble as usual, so up to the bath we went. This time the red blotches on his neck were angry. They were heaved up spots about the size of my pinky fingernail. I called for my husband to come take a look. We agreed that these were hives.

I called my good friend and a mother of three. She was more experienced than I was and once I explained what happened, she said, "Sounds like he is allergic to milk." I called the pediatrician the next morning to explain my finding. The doctor, to my surprise, made light of it and suggested trying the milk-based formula another time. But I did not. Instead, I went to our cupboard and pulled out one of the many free samples of soy formula we had received at the hospital. There was no reaction to the soy formula. From that point on I avoided milk, but not to the degree that I should have, in retrospect. I was hopeful that he would outgrow this allergic reaction at age one, as we read and were told most children do.

At the same time that we were learning about the allergies, we were moving forward on the daycare center front. Time was running out. So one summer day, out on the back deck of our new house, I wrote the deposit check. I thought that if I made the decision and got the ball rolling, the rest would fall into place and I would be on my way back to work. I hoped it was the right decision and told my husband what I'd done. He sounded surprised, "You did?" Over the next few days, we found no peace in this decision and both grew silently and increasingly uncomfortable. Each of our hearts began to sink little by little.

A few days later, when my husband was sitting at his computer, I said, "I am feeling really uncomfortable about the whole daycare thing." Without skipping a beat, he replied, "Yes, I am too." I was surprised at his clear cut response as he normally was not so opinionated. I was relieved that he felt the same as I. We talked for a short time about how uncomfortable we felt about leaving our "little fella" in daycare and about their ability to handle his dairy allergy properly. At this time, we did not know the extent or the severity of his allergies and we were assured that our son would be well cared for at the daycare center—only his own food would be given to him. We also knew how easily people can make a mistake. The daycare was a tree nut and peanut-free environment, but it allowed all kinds of dairy. We did not want our son to suffer because of a mistake made by a well meaning but busy caretaker.

In addition to our food allergy dilemma, we considered our values. By this time, the main reason for my returning to work wasn't for my fulfillment but rather for the money. To compound matters, our pediatrician surprised me one day by saying, "Why did you have a baby if you don't want to stay home and be a mom?" I was floored. Granted, I had asked him what he thought about my returning to work and leaving our son in daycare. Clearly, he didn't like the idea. Most people I have told have been shocked by his apparent political incorrectness. Even though it was shocking, I trusted this doctor. I had interviewed several pediatricians prior to having my baby and selected him because he was friendly and smiled at me. None of the other doctors smiled at me during the interviews. This doctor was an older man, perhaps in his mid-fifties, and seemed warm and kind. So when he made this statement, I felt he was really putting himself on the line for the best interest of my child. He even said, "I'm the baby's doctor—someone needs to speak for what the baby wants."

My confusion lingered as the pediatrician's words rang over and over in my mind for days and even longer. I thought, "Well, it is true that if my son is in daycare, I will see him for an hour or two in the morning and an hour or two at night, plus the weekends." Furthermore, I knew in my heart that I would be busy in the morning getting him and myself out the door, and I would be tired in the evenings. I'd probably have just enough patience and energy to feed all of us and get him to bed. The weekends would be filled with household chores and trying to make up for the time lost with my son.

So the pediatrician's "politically incorrect" advice turned out to be a powerful message to me and my heart, for which I am grateful, and a few years later, I told him so. Despite the fact that I felt we needed the money and I loved my job, I decided that staying home with my child was the right thing for us and our child. I knew it would be temporary, as the child would grow up and go to school. I would eventually return to work of some sort. We would just have to manage financially. In fact I recall reading a book that suggested selling your nice home and downsizing if it meant you could stay home with your child. At first, I didn't consider it to be realistic advice. But, in retrospect, that advice is excellent.

So about two weeks after mailing the deposit check to the daycare center, my husband and I agreed that I should remain at home to care for our son. I contacted my boss at work and set up a telephone conference call with him to tell him of our decision. After I told him, he said that he already guessed that I might not return. He was a great boss and we parted on the best of terms. I also informed the daycare center. The owner told me that the deposit was non-refundable, but it didn't matter to us because we felt confident that we were doing the best thing for our son and therefore for us.

Chapter 4: Allergy Testing

Labor Day had now come and gone. My husband and I were madly in love with our baby and thrilled about our decision for me to stay home. In fact, I felt great and our lives seemed wonderful. We were so happy that we decided we wanted another baby with whom our son could grow and play.

It was also at this time that we noticed that our son, now about eleven months old, had a chronic cough that just wouldn't quit as he played with his toys and friends. I mentioned this to my friends during play dates, and they agreed that it was unusual as their children did not cough like that. My husband grew uneasy. We had tried antibiotics, assuming that he had a bronchial infection, but it didn't change the cough. We persisted with the doctor, who decided to give me three different kinds of medication, an inhalant, an antihistamine and a decongestant. I picked up the medications unwillingly and went home.

After reading the side effects of these medications and looking at my beautiful son, who was so small and delicate, I decided that this solution was wrong and I could not pump his little body full of these medications. My husband agreed. We wanted to know why our son was coughing, not just medicate him to stop the cough.

I took my son back to the same doctor with all of the medications in hand. When the pediatrician entered the room, I said, "I don't want to give my son this medicine until we know why he is coughing." The doctor tried to convince me that the field of medicine was trial and error and often a diagnosis was made by seeing what medications were effective. I said I understood but still refused. Then he suggested that we go to an allergist. I was quite pleased with this suggestion, although a bit perplexed as to why he had not suggested this earlier.

Our son was one year old when we went to the pediatric allergist. She was a unique sort of doctor who was busily friendly and yet matter-of-fact. She brought in some toys as she explained that she would have to do a skin prick test on his back. Three sets of pricks to be exact, on three different occasions. Each appointment took about an hour, while the actual testing took twenty minutes. She explained the procedure and allergens that would be used. She said it was important that he did not touch the prick site even though it might feel itchy. Then she left to prepare the needles. The pricking of the needles didn't seem to bother him but for one second. He didn't even cry. Then the waiting started. Twenty minutes is a long time to wait while watching to prevent his back from being touched so the allergens did not smear. I glanced at the egg-timer every minute to see our progress. Twenty minutes was an eternity!

Because a one-year-old's back is fairly small, there is only enough room to place twelve pricks. The tool used looked like a plastic tray used to make home made ice pops in the freezer, except there were needles at the end of the sticks. There were two rows of prick needles, each row containing six. There has to be enough space between the pricks of allergens so that the reactions do not merge or affect each other. In other words, if the pricks are too close together, then if there is a strong reaction to one, the other, adjacent one, could be affected by appearing larger than it normally would. The pricks appeared to be about one and one-half inches apart.

The reaction sites looked like mosquito bites that are raised red lumps. Depending upon the size of the reaction, the doctor gave the allergen a level of reaction. She based it upon a scale of one through five. It appeared to me if the reaction site was about the size of a dime, then she gave it a three, a middle-of-the-road level. If it was smaller or non-existent—i.e. it just turned a bit red, but did not swell up or turn into a flat lump—then it was a one or two, or even a zero. But if it was larger than the size of a dime, she gave it a four or five. If it was bigger than the size of a quarter, then she rated it over a five, or a five plus, which is not good as it indicates a very strong reaction to the allergen.

Based upon the information that I had been given about his hives after drinking dairy formula, she did not test my son for dairy. She did not want to irritate his immune system by triggering a reaction. She explained that each time his system is exposed to the allergen his antibodies are strengthened which prolongs his ability to outgrow the food allergy. She did not test him for peanuts or tree nuts either because she did not want to trigger a new allergy by exposing him to these allergens. She said that it was likely he would have an allergic reaction to peanuts or tree nuts because he had a sensitive digestive system. She advised me not to give him any tree nuts or peanuts until he was five or six years old after his digestive system had time to mature.

The first allergen test included: cat, chicken, egg, dog, mouse, rat, dust mite, apple, banana, barley, beef, carrot and orange. The second allergen test included: ragweed, feathers, grass pollen mixes one and two, weed pollen mixes one and two, oak and birch tree, flounder, halibut, pea, potato and rice. The third allergen test included maple, tree mix, cockroach, kapok, horse, mold mixes one and two (indoor and outdoor molds), rye, soybean, tomato, turkey, watermelon and wheat.

The allergist explained that the results were negative for everything except for cat, chicken, egg and slightly for oat. She said he would probably eventually outgrow the food allergies, but that I should carry an EpiPen® Jr. and avoid those foods during the next year. She also gave me a Medic Alert form and suggested that I get a bracelet for him so others could be aware of his allergies. The prescription for the EpiPen® Jr. and suggestion for the Medic Alert bracelet shocked me.

The biggest risks, therefore, were the dairy, chicken, egg and cat. She said the chicken and egg allergy often come in pairs since eggs come from chickens. I thought about it and realized that whenever I fed him chicken dinner baby food, he would give two short coughs and a sneeze. This was amazingly consistent. We grew to recognize this reaction, which was seemingly harmless, as an allergic signal. Again, he consistently and specifically gave two short coughs in a rapid manner, and a sneeze immediately following the coughs. You could practically hear a musical beat to his reaction.

This coughing and sneezing did not seem to bother him when he was eating chicken or egg. Nor did he develop hives or red spots around his mouth when eating chicken or egg. I had rarely given him egg, only perhaps two or three times. Our pediatrician had recommended giving him some egg once he was past his first six months. So in the morning, if I cooked myself some eggs, I'd offer him a small taste. Again, I saw no reaction other than the cough, cough, and sneeze from the baby food. But as instructed, we stopped feeding him chicken and egg.

The other reaction in the testing that he had which was shocking was the strong reaction to cat dander. As described earlier, my son had been coughing for several months from about the age of eight months through ten or eleven months. We had him examined for bronchitis and the like but the pediatrician found nothing. This reaction was like a chronic hacking cough. The doctors said there was no sound of phlegm or "junk" in the lungs so it wasn't a bacterial infection such as bronchitis. Instead it was a dry cough that would affect him as he played with his toys, whether he was in our home or someone else's even if they did not have a cat.

The allergist explained that if we did not remove the cat from our home, then our son's chances of developing asthma would be great. She said that his asthma would be a lifelong ailment for him. I called my husband at work to tell him that our son was allergic to our cat. His first response was, "We are not getting rid of the cat." My husband loved the cat, as I did, and felt that it would be irresponsible to just "get rid" of an animal that no longer suited our needs. I explained that our son would develop asthma, a life threatening condition, if he was not kept from the cat's dander. I did some research on cat dander and learned it is made up of fur, urine and skin. The allergist told me that the cat's dander is in air and also attaches to the walls for six to nine months after the cat is removed. So not only were we to remove the cat, but also wipe down the walls in our home.

I posted signs locally for cat adoption and got a response. I convinced the woman how wonderful our cat was, but when the woman came to visit, she picked her up and the cat scratched her. It was disappointing to say the least. After some consideration and further attempts to find a new home for our cat of almost ten years, we decided to give it to the humane society. It was a painful process for us. My husband had a tear or two. For some reason, I was less emotional. I felt there was no contest between my son's health and the cat. Further I was pregnant and had concerns about cat feces from the litter box. My husband cleaned the litter box, but it was another point of tension for us—my husband worried about the possible affects on the fetus. Also, when I learned about the cat dander being all over our house, it really turned my stomach to think we were living with cat urine on our walls. I strongly believed we had no real choice and I could not enter into the exhausting turmoil of regret and sadness.

After returning home from dropping off our cat, I researched how to remove cat dander and other allergens from our home. I was determined to clean the house right—the first time. I found a company on the Internet that specialized in allergen cleaning and protection products. I purchased laundry detergent from them to add to my regular laundry detergent to help remove allergens from clothing and linens. I remember seeing our cat in our son's crib at times. So her dander was everywhere. I also purchased spray for dusting to capture the dander and not just spread it around. Further, I found allergen trapping vacuum bags—which trap the fine dust allergens rather than allow them to blow back out of the vacuum cleaner—that I continue to use to this day. I wiped down the walls of our home. Doing this while pregnant was exhausting. But it was all worth it because amazingly our son's chronic cough disappeared without medication, except for a few days of saline moisturizer, within two weeks of removing our cat and cleaning the walls and linens with allergen detergent.

Another consideration with my son's cough that was not explored further, because the removal of the cat worked, was cystic fibrosis testing. When I was planning my pregnancy, the blood tests showed that I was a carrier of the cystic fibrosis gene. We had my husband's blood tested as well and were happy to learn that he did not carry the same gene, thereby reducing or negating our chance of having a child who would have cystic fibrosis. Yet another alternative the allergist considered was treating my son's lung with an inhaled corticosteroid. Again, this path was not considered further because removal of the cat and her dander worked.

Someone mentioned that perhaps my house was too clean and therefore, my son developed food allergies because his immune system was just "waiting" to react to something. I considered this suggestion along with the cat allergy. Doesn't the cat allergy exist in direct contrast to this theory? Specifically, since we had a cat, wasn't my son being exposed to a "dirty" environment so that his immune system had something normal to which to respond so that he did not need to develop an allergy to foods? It didn't work out that way since he developed an allergy to both foods and the cat.

When my son turned two, he had his annual allergy test. This time, my husband took the morning off from work because I asked him to come to the appointment. I wanted him to be involved and to have the opportunity to ask questions directly to the doctor. Sometimes, he would say, "Did you ask her this or that?" and my response would be, "No." So having him at the appointment relieved me of the responsibility of asking all of his questions—ahead of time.

Our son was only tested for previously positive allergens, plus dairy. This test result indicated that he remained allergic to egg, chicken and dairy. The worst reaction was to dairy. He scored a five plus, on a scale of one to five. The welt on his back from the skin prick grew to the size of a silver dollar. The egg and the chicken were between a three and a five. I cried on the way home from the allergist's because I had hoped that he would have outgrown his dairy allergy by now, but instead it was off the charts. I remember the snowy country road was blurry from my tears.

My husband and I decided to remove all dairy and eggs from our home. We replaced the dairy products one by one. We purchased a butter substitute made mostly of canola oil. We tried soy milk instead of cow's milk. At the local health food store, I found a wonderful soy ice cream that was truly delicious. We stopped buying prepackaged foods and I got busy cooking each meal from scratch. It was not hard to cook meals from scratch. Mostly, it meant cooking longer, about one hour prior to dinnertime. All of these changes took time, effort and a positive attitude. Over about six months we completely changed our diets bit by bit. We now ate organic potatoes (roasted, mashed or baked), brown rice, meat or fish, and fresh steamed or sautéed vegetables.

We also introduced probiotics into my son's diet, from a non-dairy source, specifically a supplement. Probiotics are "good bacteria" for the digestive system such as acidophilus which is found in yogurt. We read that this might help a child outgrow his or her food allergies, although there is no proof. We gave him a tablet most mornings. I checked with the allergist, and she said that it couldn't hurt to give him the probiotics, and in fact there was some evidence that probiotics helps *prevent* food allergies. She countered by citing that there was no evidence that it helps *cure* food allergies. She also said it might help my son's digestive system mature and improve his immune system as well.

As instructed by our allergist, we brought our son in for his annual test when he turned three. She found he was no longer allergic to chicken. His dairy allergy dropped from a five-plus down to a three, on a scale of one to five. His egg allergy remained a five, which wasn't good. But in general, we were very happy with these results. Actually, I was ecstatic about the two point drop in the dairy allergy. I thought perhaps the allergist had made a mistake and confused the egg with the dairy results. So I called her to ask. But she confirmed her results were accurate.

We believed that the egg reaction remained high because of our son's vaccinations and flu shots. All of these shots were cultured in egg. Our allergist recommended that we did not give him a flu shot the next year. My husband did some research on the Internet and found an alternative to the flu shot. It was a product that could be given to our children once they had already contracted the flu. If it was given within the first forty-eight hours, this product would greatly reduce the severity of the flu. We discussed this product with our pediatrician and he gave us a prescription for the drug, so we could have some on hand if we needed it during the year. We promised our doctor that we would not use it unless he gave us the go ahead after a nasal swab test for the flu.

The allergist recommended a blood test for our son to determine if he was allergic to peanut and tree nuts. Neither she nor we wanted to administer the tests by skin prick because that would expose our son to the peanut or tree nut allergens, which could trigger an allergy. We took him to a diagnostic center and the nurse drew the blood. It was painful for our son and for us to watch. His arm was so tiny, but the nurse was skilled with children. She instructed me how to hold him while she drew his blood. Then, we received a call from our allergist with the results within two weeks. We were relieved to learn that there was no antibody present in his system for peanuts or tree nuts.

Over the next year, we continued our strict adherence to the dairy-free, egg-free home environment. We increased the probiotics (good bacteria) supplements in his diet. We believed the probiotics greatly improved his overall health and his ability to digest foods more fully, since he grew a lot that year. For more details, please see the chapter entitled, "Probiotics Are Good."

We retested our son again at age four. His egg allergy had dropped to a three (on a scale of one to five), but the dairy allergy remained at the level of three. I tried to be optimistic that we had at least made some progress on the egg allergy, but I was disappointed that we did not make any progress on the dairy allergy. I tried to console myself by pointing out that at least the dairy allergy did not become any worse.

In summary, over the four years of our son's life, we removed all dairy and egg from our diets. The biggest change occurred during our son's second year. So his environment was safe from these allergens for only eighteen months of those four years. I was pregnant with our second son before the changes to our diets were made.

CHAPTER 5: OUR SECOND SON

It was Thanksgiving and my brother's family and sister were visiting. My brother made turkey soup the night of Thanksgiving after rifling through my cabinets to see what he could find to add to the soup. It was delicious and was filled with egg pastina, carrots, celery and a lot of turkey. My sister, sister-in-law and I played cards late into the evening—it was great. I had a bowl of soup and then another. My sister and sister-in-law were laughing at me for eating and eating, all after the Thanksgiving dinner. No one yet knew I was pregnant, not even me.

Once again, while pregnant, my appetite skyrocketed. Throughout this pregnancy, I consumed dairy products, chicken, eggs and just about everything I ate during the first pregnancy. I remember eating ice cream, yogurt, pizza and milk (as we had not yet made the dietary changes in our household as described previously). I surely ate peanut butter and jelly on crackers, a favorite evening snack. I gained the forty pounds, again. The only problem that I experienced during the pregnancy was the same problem as with the first: If I did any exercise or mildly strenuous activity, my muscles would ache for days. I increased my calcium supplement under the belief that the aching muscles were a result of a need for more calcium. Much of my pregnancy was spent chasing my first son around at the park and yard. Then I'd collapse at naptime and be so grateful for the rest.

At four o'clock on a warm August morning, my water broke. I'd been out the night before with my other mommy friends having a wonderful time at our monthly dinner out. I remember laughing so hard making my big belly jiggle up and down. My regular ob/gyn was away on a biking trip, so I called the back up physician. Then I lay in bed hoping the contractions wouldn't start until my friend woke up, so I could ask her if she could take care of our son for the day. An hour later I called and asked for the favor. With great relief she obliged and we dropped our son off at seven o'clock.

Off to the hospital we went. I was hooked up to the monitors by nine o'clock and lay in the bed for about two hours with only occasional contractions. At eleven o'clock the doctor arrived and suggested that he use Patosin to speed up the contractions and the delivery. I agreed and was hooked up in seconds. Within minutes my contractions did increase in severity and frequency. Just three hours later my second son was born at nine pounds two ounces. The doctor teased, "What did you eat?" when he saw the size of my son. He had a big barrel chest, like my husband. The baby was big, healthy and absolutely beautiful. I wanted to hold him and was able to breastfeed my son almost immediately.

The nurses took him to the nursery to wash and weigh him. I learned later that they also fed him cow's milk-based formula. I was not pleased about this at all. In fact, I was quite angry, but since what had been done was done, I did not want to make a scene. Instead, I explained to them that my first son has a severe dairy allergy and I had no intention of giving my second son any dairy so as to prevent the onset of yet another allergy. They said that his blood sugar was very low, dangerously low and he really needed some food, so that is why they did it. To this day, I still feel it was wrong of them to give him the formula without checking with me first. I had made it clear that I intended to breastfeed and would have appreciated the chance to feed him myself, and if that did not work, then I would have requested they give him soy-based formula.

When I told the pediatrician this story, he calmly explained that just because one child has an allergy, it doesn't mean the sibling will have the same allergy. I know he was trying to be calming, since it already happened. The lesson to be learned is that if I were to have another child, I would tell the nurses about my children's allergies well before the child was born and make it clear what I wanted to do about his or her feeding. I did not do that and so am probably partially to blame for what happened. Despite this unfortunate incident, our second son appeared healthy, although he eventually developed dairy allergy, too—when tested at two. He breastfed with ease and was a calm and pleasant baby who seemed quite content to be held and touched.

Once we were home we told our first son, who was nineteen months old, that he received a big present: A little brother. I remember joking with my husband, "They can play together in a few months—like twelve!" We had our hands full with two young children, but we were both thrilled.

We kept our newborn son on breast milk for several months, but that was surely still tainted with dairy and eggs, since I had not yet modified my diet until later. Even so, we never directly fed him directly to chicken, eggs, dairy, peanuts or tree nuts—we fed him a diet similar to what our first son ate.

Our second son was tested for allergies at age two. He was tested only for the allergens to which his brother showed a reaction. Specifically, he was tested for chicken, egg and dairy. He was allergic to all three, but he was relatively less allergic to each than his brother was at that same age. Our second son showed a level of three for chicken and dairy, and five for egg, on a scale of one to five.

The next allergy test was done when he was three. By that point, his chicken allergy went away. The egg allergy dropped from a five to a three, on a scale of one to five. The dairy allergy remained at a three. We haven't had him tested for peanuts or tree nuts so as not to trigger and allergy, nor have we given him these foods. We are pleased that our second son has less severe allergies than our first son.

We are thankful that both boys' allergies have become less severe over the years. Our goal has been to protect their diet as much as possible now, before they enter kindergarten, so that they have the best chance of outgrowing their allergies.

CHAPTER 6: MY ALLERGY I.Q.

I admit that upon confirming with the allergist that our first son was allergic to dairy, egg and chicken, I still did not understand it nor want to believe it. I can now recall, with a measure of guilt, a string of incidents that demonstrate my lack of understanding and acceptance.

It was mid-winter, my first son was about one year and I took him to the grocery store. He was babbling in the cart seat and getting a bit squirmy. So, I gave him some cheese wrapped in plastic to hold while I shopped. As I rounded the corner of an aisle, I noticed he was coughing and coughing. His face was getting red and his eyes started to water. His coughing was violent as his head started to shake during the exhale. I stopped walking and started to panic. Did he choke on something? I looked at the cheese. He has bitten through the plastic. Was there plastic caught in this throat? Should I call the manager? Should I run with him to the car? What should I do? He coughed for about one minute then stopped abruptly.

I stood there next to the fish stand with beads of sweat all over me and realized that he probably had just had a mild anaphylactic response to eating milk protein in the cheese he was holding. His throat must have begun to swell causing him to feel like something was stuck in his throat. What a lesson I learned. I felt like an idiot for so absentmindedly handing him a hunk of cheese. I didn't call the doctor because I felt I knew what happened. But I gave myself a strong reprimand.

Nearing the end of winter, we took our son to meet some friends for dinner at the local ice cream restaurant. Nearing the end of the dinner, our son started to fidget as little children do. I handed him a plastic coffee creamer for him to play with during those last few minutes while we paid the bill. Since he was just a baby, he habitually put everything in his mouth, including this creamer. His little sharp teeth broke through the plastic covering and the creamer splashed onto his face. Within seconds he developed red spots on his face around his mouth, on his chin and onto his cheeks. I pointed this out to my friend and she was amazed at the sensitivity and speed of the reaction. The point is that if I fully understood the allergy to dairy and how counterproductive, if not dangerous, it was to expose him to dairy, then I would have never allowed him to handle the coffee creamer, or taken him to an ice cream restaurant for dinner.

In the spring, my sister visited. She brought some sour cream and onion chips. Just before we left to go shopping, my husband wanted to give our son a chip. I shrugged and said, "Okay." Neither of us thought very much about it. My son took it and ate it. It was fun watching him enjoy the new flavor—he liked it and smiled wanting more. A few seconds later when I strapped my son into the car seat, he started to cough. I ignored it at first, started the engine, and pulled out of the garage. He was still coughing so I stopped and looked at him in the rear-view mirror. I thought for a second and realized that we had just given him dairy in the chip. He was having a mild reaction. Then the coughing ceased. This incident was simply based upon us not thinking. We didn't even consider that there was dairy in the chip. It was all too new to us.

On summer evening as I made dinner, I sat our son in his highchair so that he could watch me cook while he ate. I picked up a knife that appeared to be clean since it looked shiny and unused. I cut a green grape into two pieces and gave it to my son on his highchair tray. He ate it. Within a few seconds he started coughing and red bumps appeared on his chin and near his lips. He then stopped coughing. I noticed that the knife I had used to cut the butter was gone. Actually, I had used the butter knife that I thought was clean to cut the grape into two pieces.

This time I was really angry with myself. I was beginning to realize how difficult it was to keep every bit of dairy away from him, especially if we had it in the house. Even trace amounts of allergens are dangerous as they can both trigger an allergic reaction that is visible and one that is invisible. Specifically his body could have an invisible reaction by creating antibodies to the allergen. This would delay his ability to outgrow the allergy. I concluded that I really needed to be much more careful in my practices. I should always use clean utensils in preparing his foods and if there was any doubt, then I should take a clean one out of the drawer. It did not matter that I was making more dirty dishes or utensils.

About six months later, when my son was almost two, I had a better understanding of the allergy, but think I still didn't accept it. The incident started at the local store where I picked up a bag of sour cream and onion chips (again) for myself and then a bag of plain chips for my son. We were ready to drive home. I opened his bag of chips and placed a handful of them in his lap. Then I opened my sour cream chips and ate them. About halfway home, he began clamoring for more chips. So I consciously did not wipe my hands but reached into the bag of chips for him and handed him another handful on his lap. There was a little rebellious elf sitting on my shoulder saying, "Just try it. He has probably grown out of the allergy by now and you'll make the discovery. The worry will be over and life will be good, besides, you're giving him plain chips there is just a bit of residue on your hands and it won't matter." And so hoping that I would discover his allergy was no longer a problem, I handed him chips with the sour cream dust on my fingers.

Within a few minutes we were home and he had begun to cough. I took him out of the car seat and looked at his face. His lips looked bigger than normal. I wasn't completely sure, but they did look odd. He had red spots on his face, hives. My little rebellious experiment failed. Not only did it fail, but I put my son in danger of a reaction and probably delayed his ability to outgrow the allergy. Specifically, each time the human body is exposed to the allergen, the antibodies become strengthened. The more antibodies the less chance the child has to outgrow the allergy. My lack of acceptance provoked an experiment that failed and actually caused some risk to my son's health.

If I had researched his allergy right from when we first discovered it—about six months of age—then these incidents from age one year to two years wouldn't have happened. By the time of my son's second birthday, we might have had better news, maybe not, but maybe so. Because each incident involved a tiny amount of dairy our fear grew when we wondered what a mouthful of dairy might do to him. My son's allergist had advised me to carry the EpiPen® Jr. with me wherever we went. She also suggested that antihistamine could be given as well, for a smaller reaction. My husband and I set up two packs with the EpiPen® Jr. and antihistamine we would each need to bring with our son on outings.

CHAPTER 7: OUR ACCEPTANCE

At my son's first allergy visit, I felt disbelief upon being told that our son had food allergies. As I stood in the doctor's office, she said, "No dairy, chicken or eggs for a year." I thought, "A year? That is a really long time!" I've found my feeling was not unique. Most parents report that their initial feelings are shock and disbelief. I remember *wanting* the doctor to say, "Don't worry, he'll definitely outgrow the allergy by age three." Or, "Don't worry, he can't go into anaphylactic shock from dairy." But she didn't say anything like this. If fact, she said, "Some children don't outgrow dairy until they are in early adolescence. It's really hard to say what amount and type of dairy could set him off into anaphylactic shock, so keep him away from all of it and always carry the EpiPen® Jr. Furthermore, even trace amounts of dairy will hinder his body's ability to outgrow the allergens because his antibodies will be strengthened every time he encounters the trace dairy so avoid lactic acid in bread and a variety of other hidden milk ingredients."

At the second allergy test, there was a turning point for my accepting the allergies. We went for the test, hoping that my son's allergies would miraculously be gone. But we were extremely disappointed to learn that my son's allergies were quite serious. His dairy allergy was over a five on a scale of one to five. I was still in a state of disbelief because I was angry, sad and disappointed. I was also exhausted and my eyes welled with tears on the way home. I began to imagine how our son would survive in school. I became terrified. I imagined him sitting alone at a lunch table. Everyone knows the feeling of being left out at times and I dreaded this future for our son. Something changed in my husband at that point, too. His wheels began to turn on how we could help to solve this problem. His input and participation was vital to our accepting our son's food allergies because it enabled us to make changes in our own diets so the allergens could be completely eliminated in our home.

I know other parents who have experienced the same feelings upon finishing their children's allergy testing appointments. Some moms cry in the allergist's office. Others like me cry on the way home, though I admit I felt my mouth tremble upon the final moments in the appointment. Do the allergists deal with this all the time and, therefore, develop a thick skin to the parent's emotional state? They probably do to some extent. Should the allergist help the parent? Perhaps, but it is probably unrealistic to expect her to do so due to time constraints. Once home, what can a parent do to handle the emotional state of pain, fear, and confusion?

Parents can read books, such as this one, to help them understand that they are not alone. Parents can seek out other parents in their community or on the Internet for emotional support. Schools, libraries and town clerks can be contacted to see if local support groups exist. If no local group exists, one can be created by a parent. Usually, local libraries or churches can be used as a meeting place for these groups, free of charge. A weekly or monthly meeting can be held to share stories, recipes and support.

A more private form of emotional support can be found with a counselor or therapist. Insurance companies report that most plans will cover mental health visits if properly pre-approved. A monthly visit can provide the parent some empathy and new ideas for dealing with anxiety. It is extremely important that the parents not only take care of their children, but also take care of their own feelings. If a parent's feelings are neglected, frustration and sadness could build up and affect the relationship between the parents or the parent and the child. Don't make the situation worse by treating the child with anger or disappointment. It isn't his or her fault or choice to have developed food allergies.

Parents can also take practical action by researching their child's food allergies. Preparing a detailed list of all the ingredients to which your child is allergic is an excellent first step. Allergens can be hiding behind certain names such as "arachis" for "peanuts." Parents can also purchase recipe books to learn how to provide their children with allergen-free foods. Often seeking out a health food store is necessary as well. Most of the ingredients in high profile prepackaged foods in regular grocery stores are riddled with preservatives that contain allergens or are manufactured in factories that also produce products that contain most allergens.

In retrospect, I believe that acceptance is the first step in healing. Acceptance, for us, included understanding the allergens, researching the foods we ate, and making significant changes to our family's diet. This is difficult to do overnight. It took us many months—about six to be exact. Until we fully accepted that our children have food allergies we changed neither our environment nor our thinking. Once the environment and thinking are changed, then the chance for an allergic reaction is reduced and the child's ability to outgrow the allergy is improved.

CHAPTER 8: OUR LIFESTYLE CHANGES

My husband and I were now fully cognizant of the problem. Together we totally changed our diets. We had already removed the cat and eventually removed all dairy and egg from our house. We stopped buying all take-out foods. Having dairy foods in our home meant creating a hazardous environment for our son, even if he didn't eat them. For example, our allergist told me that a dairy allergic child had a reaction at a daycare pizza party. The caretakers strapped the allergic child into a highchair and faced him to the wall. But the child broke out into hives because the cheese was hot and the proteins floated into the air. This makes sense if you consider that you can easily smell a hot pizza but not a cold one. In contrast to acceptance, there is denial. Examples of denial might be to continue eating allergy producing foods in our own home that put our children in danger or not filling our son's prescription for an EpiPen® Jr. and carrying it with us.

It took about six months to make the most significant changes. We, like many people, were addicted to cheese. But, we reluctantly stopped purchasing pizza on Friday nights and slowly eliminated our consumption of cheese on pastas and sandwiches. We started reading the ingredient lists on the foods we purchased and stopped buying foods with more than five or ten ingredients or a litany of things we didn't understand. We did such things as changing the butter that we purchased to an imitation butter made from canola oil.

We continued to get take-out food from the local Italian restaurant or the Chinese restaurant, but tried to avoid foods that contained cheese and peanuts. Even so, as we ate, our enjoyment began to fade. We began to wonder, "What exactly are we eating?" We concluded that all the Italian restaurant foods were saturated with butter and sprinkled with cheeses that would get on our fingers as we ate. Inevitably we needed to assist our son by breaking apart his food or bringing him more. So we'd have to get up and wash our hands so we would not contaminate his food. Our son would complain, as babies do, while we took this extra minute to clean our hands. This was stressful. Further, the need to wash and worry about the trace allergens on our hands would interrupt our dinner and reduce the enjoyment of our take-out food "treat."

Soon we began to realize that the take-out food wasn't a treat at all. Specifically, it was causing us stress because we had to worry and wash up so we did not spread trace allergens around our kitchen and son's food. Second, we increasingly became uncomfortable with what we were eating. The conversation at our dinner table often began to sound like, "I wonder what is in this?" Then the treat we thought we were enjoying wasn't a treat at all. It didn't decrease stress, it increased it. Plus we were paying more for it. We realized this wasn't an expense that was really buying us any enjoyment. In fact, we'd often end up in a bit of an argument by the end of the meal. So, over the six months we pretty much gave up all take-out food. If we were to eat out, it would be at a restaurant without our son and we'd wash our hands well before coming back into the house.

This level of acceptance put us on the right track. Now we were well on our way to a dairy-free environment in our own home for our son's sake. The good news was that not only were we doing the right thing for our son's health, but our stress levels went down because the tension of trace allergens, washing and tracking what we ate or touched was no longer an issue. The elimination created a sort of safe haven in our own home.

After a short time, we did not miss those foods very much. Perhaps seeing a pizza commercial caused us the most desire, but a commercial ends after a few seconds. In contrast, the peace of mind we gained by eliminating those foods gave us relief. We relaxed because we knew we were doing the right thing for our children in the short and long term. We were freed from our feelings of guilt.

The freedom that we experienced was from the nagging feeling that we weren't being honest with ourselves. By pretending that exposing our son to food allergens wouldn't matter, there had been guilt that we weren't doing our absolute best as parents. We were being a little selfish when we still purchased butter or ate a pizza in our own home or in the presence of our children. It made us uncomfortable and often ruined the enjoyment of the meal, especially when our son asked for a taste of what we were eating. The sacrifice of the foods that we liked turned out not to be a sacrifice at all. Instead, it was a gift that we could give to our children. Sacrificing those foods, for their sake, was an easy thing to do after a little practice.

There was one other huge benefit to our acceptance and change: Our own diets improved. We looked at every ingredient list of the foods that we purchased. We bought only those items that contained five or less ingredients that we *understood*. In other words, we stopped eating a lot of preservatives found in commercial breads, cookies, crackers and other foods that have a long shelf life. Instead we increased our consumption of fresh breads, whole grain pastas, brown rice, organic potatoes, fruits and vegetables.

My husband who is about six feet tall had been a bit overweight. He is a computer software engineer and did not get a lot of exercise during the day. He started swimming once a week for about an hour. Coupled with that change was the change we made to our diet and the elimination of all dairy. Within six months by husband lost about fifty pounds. He looked like a new person and felt like a new person. He was happy. He had more energy and could move with ease. In short, our acceptance of our son's food allergy affected us in ways we could never have imagined.

Once a parent fully accepts the allergy and makes it his or her own, there is a wonderful feeling of freedom. Once the allergens are identified and removed from the child's home a sense of control is restored. Strangely, with that control, freedom is created. When we removed all food allergens from our house and took steps to prevent exposure to food allergens outside the house we felt better. We knew in our hearts that we were doing the best we could to enable our children to outgrow their food allergies. We reminded each other and ourselves that whatever happened in the future, we are doing the best we can now.

Another step we took was to advise babysitters and friends that we kept a dairy-free home. A new babysitter would often thank me after I told her this before she came over, while we were on the telephone. I would always tell her that she is welcome to eat anything she might like in our home just please don't bring snacks in. She was glad to know the situation and the fact that we were forthright about it.

We did the best we could and tried to maintain a balance in our social lives by not living in a bubble. We avoided environments that were surrounded by food and were dangerous. For instance, we would not take our children to fast food restaurants nor let them play in those areas which would undoubtedly be covered with trace amounts of food allergens.

Additionally, we did not take our children on airplanes because if they were to have an allergic reaction there would be no way to get them to a hospital since it would require an emergency landing of the airplane. A pilot friend of mine told me that a plane cannot do an emergency landing in less than one hour. Since each EpiPen® Jr. dose lasts for only twenty minutes, I figured that we could give two doses to cover forty minutes of a reaction, which might not be enough. So we gave up visits to our children's grandparents and aunts, who live too far for us to drive there. We visited family by auto only. We were not willing to take the risk of flying.

We will consider air travel in the future but will do so carefully. We will research security laws for flights to determine what foods we can bring onto the plane. Since we cannot purchase food at the airports, we will have to plan and pack all of the foods our children and we will need. We will also have to plan where we will purchase the foods once we are at our destination. This means researching the location of health food stores ahead of time, or even giving our relatives a list of foods and brand names of foods that will work for our children. Taking these steps is helpful to reduce the stress in traveling.

Up to this point in time, the cumulative effects of taking all of these preventative measures caused my husband and me too much stress to be worth the trip. For this reason, we decided that spending money on a vacation that would be stressful isn't fun. So we did not want to do it. Our solution was to ask the children's relatives to come and visit us or to make shorter trips by car. We just had a visit from the children's grandmother a few days ago. Everyone had a wonderful time. I'd even consider offering to pay or partially pay for the plane fare, if a relative wanted to visit but couldn't afford it. It is worth the peace of mind and freedom from worry, stress, and exhaustion.

As part of accepting the seriousness of the food allergy, I found it important to take care of myself, too. As a primary caregiver to these children, there was little break time. One important outlet for me was to join a health club that had a food-free and drink-free child watch room. When our son was three months old I looked in the yellow pages of the phone book for health clubs. To my surprise and joy, the advertisement for a couple of health clubs within twenty minutes driving distance offered child care.

I immediately called the health club to see if this was true. Indeed it was. Upon visiting the club, I was apprehensive about leaving my child with someone else, especially in the room with other children. My mother suggested leaving my baby in his car seat and bringing the stroller in so that he would be high up off the ground and away from other children's sneezes and hands. This was an excellent idea. There were several caretakers in the room watching the children and a sign on the door that states, "No food or drink allowed." Also, I told the manager of the child watch room that my son had food allergies to dairy, egg and chicken. She assured me that he would be safe.

Despite the assurances and adult supervision, there was one time, several years later, when I came back from exercising and saw my younger son, when he was about one year old, holding a bottle of formula just about to drink some. I took the bottle from him and asked the caretakers whose bottle it was, because my son had food allergies. One woman admitted it was hers and indeed had milk-based formula in it. Although I felt angry and startled, I calmed down and explained how serious my children's reactions could be. The supervisors were interested in hearing the details and asked several questions in response. I answered their questions and realized I should have explained in more detail earlier.

Upon getting home, I called my husband at work to tell him what had happened. I was afraid he would become upset and suggest that I not return to the health club. At this point, the health club was something I needed for my own care, both for mental health and physical health as it provided me a break from household chores for a few hours each week. But instead my husband's response was to suggest that we call the general manager and explain what happened. We agreed and he called. He later told me that he explained to her about the trace amounts of allergen that could be found in foods, so many foods not apparently dairy, could be a threat to our children. He further mentioned that the health club could have liability issues, i.e. could be sued, if a child came to harm through food allowed in the child watch room, even though the sign on the door stated that no food was allowed. Surely, this had an impact on her and she admitted there had been an incident previously and they should adhere more carefully to their own rule.

The response was that the child watch supervisors held meetings to explain the seriousness of not allowing food or drinks in the child watch room. They began to enforce their own rule more carefully. The caretakers seemed more aware when we reminded them that our children had food allergies. They would smile and assure us that they would be careful. Occasionally, when we dropped off our children we would notice that a supervisor had a cup of coffee on the counter top. When this occurred we would mention our children's allergy to dairy and inquire if they had cream in their coffee. They would usually respond that they would be careful with the coffee and we would let it go at that. At a minimum it served as a reminder to them that our children had food allergies and that we were aware of the no food no drink rule, and that it was being bent. To this day, about two years later, there has not been another incident in the child watch room with respect to our children coming into contact with food or drink. Despite the incident, the health club is an excellent way to take care of a mother. It gives the children some time to play with new toys and make some friends in a food-free room, where the parent is close by in case of an emergency or a diaper change.

In summary, we changed our lifestyle to eliminate food allergens from our home. This helped to reduce our stress levels. We also found that these changes improved our own diets because we were paying more attention to the ingredients in the foods we ate. We also enriched our lifestyle by joining a health club for exercise and further stress reduction. We tried to maintain things we enjoyed in a way that would not harm our children, such as when we dined out with friends we'd be careful not to bring any trace food allergens home on our clothes or hands. In short, our lifestyle was changed for the better due to our children's food allergies.

Other Parents' Stories

INTRODUCTION

I thought it would be interesting to learn and share other parents' stories for the purpose of this book so that you could read about a variety of experiences, attitudes and solutions. I have found this process to be fascinating, exhilarating and exhausting. Most of the interviews were conducted in the presence of our children as they played together. The children would interrupt us numerous times while the story was told. It was noisy, fun and exciting for everyone involved.

I was most affected by the emotion as the mothers told their stories. Some mothers cried, others felt goose bumps or anger as they recalled and explained a particularly troublesome time in their experiences of discovering that their child had a food allergy. Some mothers took a deep breath during the hard memories. Almost every mother expressed frustration with their doctors by stating that they did not feel listened to with enough compassion or get enough help identifying the food allergies as quickly as perhaps they should have.

I listened carefully as I scribbled hand-written notes. I remember getting goose bumps on my arms or the back of my neck feeling the intensity of the mother's pain, fear or anger. Sometimes a big lump would grow in the back of my throat and my eyes would water a bit. After each interview, I would be emotionally drained and could not stop thinking about the mother's story for the next few days. Because of this, I could only conduct two interviews a week at the most. I was also apprehensive before some interviews fearing that the child might come into contact with some food to which he or she is allergic in my home. This was a new perspective for me since normally I was the only parent with the allergic children. Other times I woke up at night remembering an interview and feeling scared for children especially when they are to enter school with a peanut allergy.

Most of the interviews were of families who live in the United States. But some of the families live in other countries or were raised in other countries. I wanted to learn if this silent epidemic is affecting the United States more severely than in other countries. I found the problems associated with food allergic children tend to be the same, regardless of where the family lives. At the end of this section is a chapter that summarizes the major food allergens, labeling laws and any statistics for sufferers of food allergies in countries around the world. These statistics show that many developed countries are suffering from food allergies in their children.

Some of the parent's and children's names have been changed upon their request. All of the parents were happy to share their story and their advice. Most wanted to be sure that the readers understood how important it is to be confident when dealing with relatives, doctors and caretakers. Many shared how they felt it important to read about food allergies and keep a positive attitude.

Chapter 9: Karen's Story

Karen is a forty-year-old mother of two. She is a vigilant and energetic mother of a nine-month-old and a two-year-old. She lives in the United States. At the park, she watches her children carefully as the other mothers sit or chat nearby. Prior to having children she worked as a clinical social worker. Now she is a full-time mother working long hours in her own home.

Her son Max is just over two years. When her daughter was born, Max was twenty months. It was at that time that Karen began to suspect that Max had food allergies. She has since learned that he is highly allergic to peanuts, walnuts and cashews and also allergic to egg, wheat, dust mites, horse hair, and trees. Max also has extremely sensitive skin and will develop a red mark or hive through contact with cold ice cream, a rough beard, tomato sauce and even a strong grip of a loving hand.

It all started when a friend suggested that Karen give Max peanut butter to supplement his protein intake, which was advice that the friend had been given by a pediatrician. Karen was concerned about Max's protein intake because he did not like to eat meat. Karen was aware that peanut allergies could be severe and was somewhat concerned. Initially, she decided to give him some peanut butter while they were at the hospital just after the birth of Karen's second child, her daughter. She felt that it would be a safe place to expose him. It might not have been the first time that Max had come into contact with peanuts. Perhaps he picked up some peanut shells that his parents were eating when they went camping. Further, he probably ate ice cream that has a peanut butter swirl in it. But he never showed a reaction.

A couple of months later when Max was ill with a cold, Karen gave him a peanut butter cracker to munch along with a bit of apple. The peanut butter was chunky style. About five minutes later Max vomited. Karen recalls, "I wasn't sure if this was a reaction to the peanut butter or if it was just a normal reaction for a child who had a lot of mucus from his cold since he had been vomiting occasionally during his cold. Maybe the chunky pieces in the peanut butter got caught in his throat or mixed with the apple in a way that made him feel like he was gagging, thereby causing him to vomit. I just wasn't sure."

Shortly after vomiting, it was time for Max's nap. Karen noticed that he had puffy eyes and a slight rash around his mouth when he woke up. The puffy eyes were unusual for Max, but the slight rash was not. Max had extremely sensitive skin and often had red marks or small rashes just from touch. Karen took note of these signs with some concern. She discussed her concerns with her husband, who felt that Karen was overreacting and there was nothing to worry about.

The next day, Karen called Max's pediatrician. When she spoke with the nurse about these signs that Max had, the nurse replied, "If he has a peanut allergy it is serious and can be fatal." Karen was devastated, not only with this news, but by how the nurse handled the situation in making this presumption and stating the horror associated with it. The nurse gave Karen the name of an allergist, whom Karen called immediately and with much emotion. Karen remembers, "I felt hysterical and the allergist must have sensed that because he offered to see Max that same day."

Karen, her mother and husband took Max to the allergist together where he underwent a skin prick test of roughly sixteen allergens. When the results were in, the allergist reported that Max was allergic to peanuts, walnuts, cashews, egg and wheat and a few other environmental non-food allergens. Karen was distraught and started to cry. "I couldn't believe what was happening," she painfully recalls. "I knew of the seriousness of food allergies since I'd worked in a preschool as a social worker," she said.

With tears in her eyes, she pleaded for some explanation or support. The allergist did not provide any but rather responded with a matter-of-fact, "We diagnose this kind of thing all day, every day." This nonempathetic response only served to send Karen further into despair. Karen was then perplexed when the allergist said, "Allergies are genetic but not inherited." She went home feeling alone and beyond sad. She remembers that day and describes it as being one of the worst days of her life. Tears again begin to fall during her retelling of the story and a lump grew in my own throat as I listened.

While caring for her two small children, one just a couple of months old, Karen began to wonder if there were any signs along the way that she missed. She considered her families' histories. Her side of the family has no food allergies at all. Her husband recalls that his father had rough elbows, but don't a lot of people? He also recalls that his grandmother had eczema at times. Other than that, Karen's husband reacted strongly to a bee sting once. Karen further considered what she ate during her pregnancy and breastfeeding months. Not being a big meat eater, she would supplement her protein intake with a peanut butter and jelly sandwich a couple of times a week. "Could that have contributed to it?" she wondered.

Karen recalls that Max, around four months of age, had eczema. When she discussed it with the two dermatologists neither one mentioned food allergies as a possible cause. Instead they only prescribed cream. Later, when Karen asked them why they didn't mention food allergies they said that so many people have eczema and they can't tell everyone who has eczema that it could be related to food allergies. "Shouldn't they at least advise me?" Karen thought.

Aside from the fact that her son does have a serious reaction to peanuts, the other major difficulty for Karen is the lack of support she feels from those around her. She and her husband often have conflicting views on how to protect her son from an accidental ingestion of peanuts. For instance, just a few days earlier, Karen's husband wanted to stop for ice cream at the local stand. Karen was concerned that the ice cream could have traces of peanut in it. Her husband said, "Don't worry, live life." But Karen said, "The experience was full of anxiety for me."

Another example of contention is during the holiday season while at her mother-in-law's house one relative brought a plate of peanut butter cookies. Karen asked everyone not to eat them because the crumbs could fall to the floor and Max could ingest them. Rather than agreeing, her mother-in-law said, "We'll just put them in the kitchen and eat them in there." Karen was angry. Peanut could still fall to the floor in the kitchen, plus peanut traces would be on the fingers and lips of anyone who ate them and then might touch or kiss Max. She says, "I felt unsupported by my husband as well because when I told him what his mother said, he didn't confront her."

She understands that her husband's lack of support is because he does not want Max to suffer socially. He doesn't want Max to feel different or be socially isolated. Karen explains, "I read about a local mother in the paper whose son appears traumatized by his peanut allergy. His mother describes his behavior to include biting his nails uncontrollably because he is so worried he will come into contact with peanuts. His mother has even tried to get his school to ban peanuts, but they will not. I certainly don't want Max to feel this nervousness, but there must be some middle ground between dangerous laxness and overprotective nervousness." Karen is reading books and highlighting passages that she will ask her husband to read with the hope that they can reach a middle ground for handling Max's food allergies.

Karen is not only concerned about Max's level of anxiety, but her own, as well. She explained that anxiety can affect her whether she is at the park or a birthday party. Karen recalls, "I recently was at the park and bought a lollipop for Max at the hot dog stand. Then I considered if there might be peanut trace in the lollipop and decided not to give it to him. Max wanted it and became upset—which made me feel just terrible. The park also poses the problem of other children walking around eating peanut butter and jelly sandwiches or granola bars. I have asked those children's mothers not to allow their children to walk around with peanut-based foods, but I feel their annoyance rather than any compassion. Also, at some birthday parties where relatives visit, I have had to ask my relatives not to drink from the same straw or eat from the same spoon as Max. These situations are becoming more frustrating for me—then my level of anxiety and anger increase because of how others treat my feelings."

Knowing that she is not alone by talking with other mothers about food allergies is the only way Karen is getting through this situation. She is also starting a local food allergy support group. She consoles herself that Max's recent scores on the RAST blood test show moderate level of reaction to peanut. She hopes that the Duke study in which exposure to small amounts of peanuts on a daily basis might help to cure a peanut allergy will succeed. She further hopes that the FDA will approve a vaccine to cure food allergies in the next five or six years. She does feel comforted by the fact that Max's egg and wheat allergies are mild and appear to be disappearing. In fact, the allergist suggested doing an "egg challenge" soon in which Max will be given egg in a controlled environment with medical staff ready to handle a reaction. Her last line of defense is to carry the EpiPen® Jr. wherever Max goes.

CHAPTER 10: JENNIFER'S STORY

Jennifer is a thirty-year-old mother of two boys William, age two, and Ethan, age five. She is bright and speaks effortlessly. She lives in the United States. Prior to having children she worked in human resources. She was adopted as a child and although she has no food allergies herself, she was advised that her biological parents had many food allergies including eggs, dairy, wheat, seafood, nuts, oranges, hair, fur, cats and dogs.

Jennifer first gave Ethan, her eldest, yogurt when he was about one year old. It didn't go well, as he broke out in hives shortly after. She continued to breastfeed him until he was thirteen months old and then introduced him to cow's milk. That did not go well either. He started to vomit right away and continued to vomit for weeks, even though she immediately stopped the cow's milk and switched to soy milk. He was also having diarrhea.

A few months later, Jennifer's mother and mother-in-law encouraged her to give Ethan some egg. Although Jennifer was skeptical of this advice, she tried the egg. Ethan broke out in terrible hives and began to vomit profusely. She recalls, "I immediately gave him antihistamine and ran a shower to fill the room with steam which I thought would calm his vomiting. After about one hour of sitting in the steamy bathroom, Ethan stopped vomiting. I don't take my mother's or my mother-in-law's advice any more."

When she took him to the pediatrician, he told her that Ethan probably just had a virus. Jennifer felt the doctor wasn't interested in exploring the possibility that her son had food allergies. But she *insisted* that he refer her to a specialist for some testing.

It took about six weeks to get an appointment with the gastrointestinal specialist to which the doctor referred her. Jennifer remembers, "Ethan was still vomiting every day and was about fifteen months old.

By now, his esophagus was so raw that it was probably causing him to continue to vomit. The doctor had Ethan drink barium so that he could x-ray him to determine if Ethan had a weak sphincter. The procedure was traumatic for Ethan and me. I had to hold him down to get him to drink the solution. After all that, they found no problems with his sphincter and prescribed Zantac®, an antacid."

Three months later, when Ethan was eighteen months, the doctors thought perhaps Ethan had celiac disease, which is an intolerance to gluten. To test this theory, they needed to take a biopsy of his intestines. They warned Jennifer that since he was still vomiting it could cause him to aspirate which could lead to death. Jennifer easily made the decision not to do the test, stating, "No test that risks my son's life is worth it."

Also at eighteen months, the doctor referred her to an allergist. Almost a year had passed since Ethan first experienced the digestive problems. In retrospect, Jennifer wishes she'd been referred to an allergist much sooner. At the appointment, she learned that Ethan was allergic to egg, dairy, wheat, tree nuts and peanuts. Even though he was slightly allergic to wheat, she did give him bread containing some wheat and found that if the bread was highly processed then the wheat did not negatively affect him.

Eventually, the vomiting quieted. Jennifer continued to give Ethan Zantac® but felt uncomfortable about giving this drug to him for such a long period of time. Unfortunately, although the vomiting improved, the diarrhea did not as Ethan approached twenty months. The doctors directed her to collect his stool for five days. Then a laboratory could analyze the stool to determine if Ethan was absorbing fats. They found he was absorbing fats and instructed her to give him breads to try to bind him up and reduce the diarrhea. Jennifer recalls that, "Ethan's allergy symptoms did not go away for some time after eliminating the offending foods, which seems to be different from what other people have experienced."

From age two to three, Jennifer studiously avoided all ingredients that contained egg, dairy, tree nuts and peanuts. She recalls only a few mistakes in which Ethan once ate a birthday cake containing egg. Another time Jennifer was making brownies and Ethan reached up and touched the raw egg in the batter, she describes, "Ethan walked from the kitchen into the family room and started to break out in hives and vomit. He didn't even eat the egg, but just touched it." Anther incident occurred in preschool, she remembers, "During his first month, the instructors accidentally handed him a cookie that contained egg. Ethan took one bite before they said they realized their mistake. A bit later, while out on the playground, Ethan started vomiting all over himself."

At age three, Ethan underwent another allergy test. Jennifer was pleased to learn that he was no longer allergic to dairy, wheat, tree nuts or peanuts. He was still allergic to eggs and cat dander and remains so at age five. Ethan is aware of his allergy and will ask his mother if a new food has egg in it or if he can eat it. If he does eat eggs, he will get a runny nose and hives.

Jennifer's two-year-old son, William, has shown positive for allergies to dairy and egg. She hasn't exposed him to either of these two foods and he has never had any adverse reactions to any foods. Her husband accidentally gave him some walnuts in a salad one time, but there was no reaction thankfully. William doesn't vomit regularly or have loose stools either and has even had cow's milk without any adverse effects.

When Jennifer first learned of Ethan's food allergies, she did not feel devastated as many mothers do. She described the feeling as being "agitated." Her son had suffered for an entire year, from age one to two, before she knew why her son was vomiting and having diarrhea. In retrospect, she says, "I wish someone could have told me right away that Ethan had food allergies. Perhaps doctors should run a standardized test at six months of age on all children to determine if they have or are prone to food allergies. I even discussed this idea with my son's doctor, but he replied that many children might have false positives and cause unnecessary worry. I disagree and think any information is useful."

Since learning about her older son's food allergies over the past two years, Jennifer has kept a positive attitude by reminding herself that her son's allergies are just part of their life. It could be worse...such as having a learning disorder, a disability, a severe latex allergy or a life threatening illness. To deal with the food allergies she vigilantly watches the ingredient list of foods that he consumes and avoids all allergens. She tries to not traumatize her son and make him fearful of food. She doesn't like limiting his diet but has done so as required. She finds Ethan to be tentative to try new foods now, especially when those foods contain ingredients to which he was previously allergic.

CHAPTER 11: LARISSA'S STORY (GERMANY/RUSSIA)

Larissa is a thirty-five-year-old mother of a three-and-a-half-year-old adorable girl. Larissa was born in Germany near Berlin and raised in Russia close to Moscow. Her father was in the military so her family moved around in Russia during her childhood. Her concerned and serious nature emanates from beneath her short blond hair and light aqua eyes. She studied chemistry, as it was her passion during her adolescence, and eventually earned her degree in chemistry. Before she had her daughter she worked as a paralegal.

Ina, her daughter, is quick and bright. She came to our interview with a little smile and was dressed in a pink and white polka dot top, white pants with bows under the knee, white socks edged with lace that where carefully folded over, and two bright pink bows in her hair that matched her bright pink clogs.

Larissa explains, "Ina is highly allergic to egg and also is allergic to shellfish, tree nuts, peanuts and cocoa. She is allergic to soy as well, but the skin prick tests could not successfully be administered because the results were so strong that the bumps spread into each other and it was impossible to tell to which allergen she is reacting." Larissa has been trying to have Ina blood tested to confirm the skin test results.

Larissa didn't give egg to her daughter until after she was one year old. Larissa remembers, "When I finally fed her the egg, Ina developed hives within two minutes of the first time she ate it. I told her doctor of the reaction, who only advised me not to give her any more egg for one year. He did not prescribe an EpiPen® Jr. nor did he recommend an allergy test."

After the year, Larissa recalls an incident at a birthday party, "Ina sat next to the cake that was covered in raspberries. I watched Ina touched the cake and then touch her face. She did not eat the any, but broke out in hives on her face and body just from touching the cake, which contained some egg. I called the on-call pediatrician who advised me to give her antihistamine. The antihistamine calmed the hives, but when the dose wore off after a few hours, the hives returned. This reaction continued for a week." After the week passed, Larissa was advised to take Ina to see an allergist. It took two months to get her daughter in for an initial appointment with the allergist.

At the appointment the test results produced a swelling for each of the allergens that were larger than a silver dollar. Since the pricks are only about two inches apart from each other, each test site was affected by its neighboring test site, making it impossible to ascertain the correct individual results. Based upon this unreadable result, the allergist recommended that Larissa have a blood test done on her daughter.

Over the past several months, Larissa has brought her daughter to a blood drawing center five or six times. Each time has proved unsuccessful. Specifically, each time a nurse has tried to draw blood Ina's tiny vein cannot be pierced. To make matters worse, the amount of blood needed to test for all the allergens is large. Each nurse is skeptical of drawing that much blood from such a young patient. As can be expected, Ina is now frightened of going to the doctors. She complains, "They make holes in my arm."

I came upon Larissa and her daughter one morning at a doctor's office. We chatted and she told me she'd been waiting for forty-five minutes. After a few more minutes she was called. Then, upon entering the blood drawing room, she learned that the nurse would not draw blood from a child and that she'd need to go to yet another blood drawing center. Larissa was amazingly calm. She accepted this information without showing any frustration or anger. I was impressed by how gracefully she handled yet another disappointment. Later, at a chance meeting, Larissa told me, "Several months later, the doctors were finally able to draw the blood and perform the test. It confirmed Ina's allergies to all the allergens in the skin prick test, except for cocoa for which they did not test."

Larrissa readily admits the strain she feels despite her calm demeanor. She recalled a particularly hard time when she first learned the extent of her daughter's food allergies. She says, "It felt like I was hit over the head. I was devastated by the news." To make matters worse, two days later her in-laws, who she'd met only once before, came to visit for six weeks. So she recalls, "Not only did my husband and I have to deal with understanding the food allergy, but we struggled and were burdened with trying to explain the seriousness of it to his parents." The seafood allergy is serious—recently, Larissa brought Ina to an aquarium, but Ina broke out in hives the minute she entered the building. They immediately left.

Larissa is frustrated and feels a great deal of stress about her daughter's food allergies. She is confused by the fact that while her daughter can eat potatoes, carrots, onion and chicken each separately, but when these same ingredients are combined into a hot or cold soup, she breaks out in hives. Larissa also admitted, "I feel others might think I am a bit paranoid about the whole thing." She responded to her own thought with, "But how can't I help do the best for my child? What would happen to her if she ingested something and had a terrible reaction?" Larissa explains, "I feel I must take each day minute by minute. I am not always sure what to do next and am concerned about what will happen when Ina goes to school for a full day."

Currently, Ina attends preschool three days a week for two and one-half hours each day. Larissa searched out schools that were most supportive of handling food allergies. The school she chose permits Larissa to provide all of her daughter's food. They promised not to give her any snacks that were not provided by her mother. Larissa was further comforted by the fact that the daughter of the school's director also has food allergies, so the responsiveness and understanding of the school appeared to be better than at others.

Responsiveness is imperative since reactions can occur and are unpredictable. One night, upon the advice of the on-call pediatrician,

Larissa brought her daughter to the emergency room because she was coughing and her face was turning red. Upon arriving at the hospital, Larissa was told to go to the waiting room. Three hours later, her daughter had still not been admitted. Larissa was beyond despair and decided to leave the hospital since her daughter's coughing had stopped. She says, "Several weeks later the hospital still managed to send a bill. No service had been administered, no doctor was seen, but a bill was sent. It was unbelievable."

Another unbelievable fact that Larissa learned is that some states don't allow the administration of an EpiPen® Jr. in an ambulance. Thankfully, her state of residence does allow it, but this does bring up the risk when traveling out of state or country. Perhaps one should check with each state to learn if EpiPen® Jr. can be administered by emergency paramedics.

Although Larissa and her husband are from Russia, they have no immediate plans to return to visit their families. They fear the plane ride. The peanut allergy makes air travel especially loathsome. Thus far their Russian families have made the trip to the United States to visit their granddaughter about once a year. Fear surrounds not only air travel, but restaurant outings as well.

Larissa and her husband rarely go out to eat anymore. They have found two restaurants where one meal at each has been safely given to their daughter. One is a Mexican place where they purchase a dish of rice and beans for their daughter. The other is of Italian specialty where they purchase a white pizza for their daughter. Otherwise, when they do dine out, they bring their daughter's dinner prepared at home ahead of time.

Larissa ponders why her beloved daughter has these allergies. She was careful during her pregnancy to exercise and eat healthy foods. She did not drink alcohol and has never smoked. "Why me?" she wonders. There was no history of food allergies in her family, except for an uncon-firmed mild egg sensitivity on her husband's side. Larissa accepted the regular childhood vaccinations for her daughter but now wonders, "Since these vaccines are cultured in egg, could this have contributed to the egg allergy?" Ina only received a flu shot once. That time, the doctors administered it with the EpiPen® Jr. in-hand should she have an allergic reaction.

Larissa further considered the fact that in Sweden and Finland children have high allergies to fish, and similarly many Japanese children are allergic to rice. Could it be that too much of one food causes allergies? Or perhaps it is the amount of chemicals and processing that is done to our food. She recalls her grandparents lived off the land and grew their own food. "Perhaps we need to get back to basics," she says.

CHAPTER 12: HEATHER'S STORY

Heather is a thirty-seven-year-old mother of three children aged five and younger. She lives in the United States. Her smile reflects her good health and lifestyle. She eats organic foods whenever possible and her husband raises pigs and chickens on their fresh-air property on a wooded hilltop.

Heather's children each have a little twinkle in their eye. Even her son, who has the most severe allergies, is big and strong at four years. He is highly allergic to wheat and dairy. Her daughter, age five, is allergic to wheat. Her youngest, a girl, has not yet shown any allergies during her one and one-half years.

When her second child, Adam, was born, Heather nursed him. At this time Heather was eating dairy and wheat, as most people do. Heather remembers the first incidents, "When Adam was about six weeks, I was nursing him while he was on his side. I noticed that his lips were turning blue, so I picked him up. Within about five seconds, he vomited like mad. I was so scared."

Shortly after, there was another incident. Heather explains, "I was bathing Adam in the kitchen sink. I had just made a snack of cheese and crackers for my daughter and was nibbling on the cheese myself. I finished bathing him and placed him in a seat. He began to vomit a sort of bubbly, frothy vomit that kept rolling out of his mouth. He also started to cough or choke. I called 911 and was so relieved when the ambulance arrived within minutes. I got into the ambulance with my kids, but by the time we got to the hospital, Adam stopped choking." She explained that the doctors did not know why Adam had been choking and she was sent home without any answers.

Heather breastfed Adam and gave him soft solid foods as well. She consumed wheat and dairy in her own diet, and thus her breast milk contained these proteins. She also fed Adam cottage cheese and yogurt.

He seemed to enjoy both of these foods a lot and did not appear to have a negative reaction to them, most of the time.

The next incident occurred when Adam was between three or four months. Heather had a dentist appointment. She says, "I fed Adam some yogurt at my home then drove to my mom's house so she could watch the kids for me. When I got to the dentist's, they told me I had a phone call. I was surprised, but answered the phone and it was my mom. She said Adam had been vomiting since I left and I should come back right away." When Heather arrived at her mother's, Adam was still vomiting and he was a horrible color of grey.

She rushed Adam to the emergency room. He had now been vomiting for about one-half hour. Once at the emergency room, the vomiting ceased. Heather says, "I felt like the staff thought I was a bit crazy." The doctor suggested that her son had acid reflux and prescribed him some medication. Heather gave it to Adam for two days. She didn't like the idea. After all, this wasn't a regular occurrence, it didn't make a lot of sense and she didn't like giving her four-month-old prescription medication.

The fourth incident occurred when Adam was about six or seven months. Heather was planning a trip to the library and as usual gave her son cottage cheese, which he enjoyed. Once at the library, Adam vomited on the floor. Heather was distraught. The librarian told her not to worry about the mess. Heather immediately picked up Adam and brought her two children to the car. She says, "I buckled Adam into his car seat and saw his eyes roll to the back of his head!"

Heather called his pediatrician from the car in the library parking lot. The pediatrician told her to go to the emergency room. Heather was terrified since each of the three closest hospitals were at least a twenty-minute drive, without traffic. She explained this problem to the doctor who then agreed to see Adam at his office, just a few minutes away.

When they arrived, Adam was still vomiting a sort of bubbly, frothy vomit. The doctor actually saw Adam's reaction this time, which provided Heather with a sense of satisfaction and relief. Up until that point, she was feeling that medical personnel thought, "I was just an over-reactive, frantic mother."

The pediatrician decided that Adam should undergo some testing at Hartford's Children's Hospital. It took about three to four weeks to get Adam in for an appointment. Once there, two tests were run. One test was to determine if Adam had an obstruction in esophagus and the other test was run to see if he was prone to seizures.

Heather reluctantly handed over her baby. The nurse gave him a bottle of barium so that the technician could x-ray his digestive tract and determine if he had any obstructions for deformities that might be causing him to vomit so profusely. The doctors thought that Adam might have a deformity of the cardiac sphincter, the valve at the top of the stomach, but the test found no deformities.

The other test run was equally traumatic for both mother and son. The doctors thought Adam might be prone to seizures. To set one off, they placed him in a strobe light. But first they placed electrodes all over his head so that they could track any brain functioning should a seizure occur. Heather recalls, "I watched the doctor put these electrodes all over my baby's head—it was terrible." The test produced no seizures, no results. Heather was sent home without answers, once again.

At Adam's eighteen month doctor's appointment the doctor examined Adam and all appeared to go well, nothing too unusual, except Adam was now experiencing some severe eczema. At the end of the appointment, Heather remembered something she'd been concerned about, so said, "Oh, also, I wanted to mention that Adam's bowel movements are usually really smelly and I normally have to give him a bath afterward." The doctor replied, "Well he probably has a dairy allergy." Heather was shocked.

The shock was from the sudden realization that perhaps this allergy led to the profuse vomiting attacks and emergency room visits over the past eighteen months. In addition to shock, Heather was angry that no one had suggested the possibility of a food allergy prior to now—eighteen months of life. She says, "My anger was lessened because I knew the situation was complicated since Adam was able to eat dairy often without a reaction. It was only once in a while that a severe reaction occurred, perhaps when the allergen built up enough in his tiny body. But still, I wish the doctors had at least mentioned the possibility of a food allergy, especially in light of the eczema."

It was then that Heather decided to go to a different type of doctor. She decided to go to a naturopathic doctor. Naturopaths heal by using herbs, supplements and other natural remedies to allow body to heal itself. As for allergies, a naturopath diagnoses using a process called kinesiology. Heather's new doctor tested both Adam and her for food allergies by having them hold unlabeled vials of allergens in their hands and testing their muscle strength.

Heather recalls, "I was amazed at my own experience and from watching Adam's reaction to the test, especially since he had no idea what he was doing or for what he was being tested." The naturopathic doctor found the results to be clear for both Heather and her son. The results demonstrated that both she and Adam were allergic to wheat and dairy. Adam's allergies were severe for wheat and strong for dairy. The doctor recommended acidophilus, cod liver oil, and a homeopathic supplement, called pulsatilla.

As instructed, Heather gives Adam, acidophilus—a beneficial bacteria that lives in the gastro-intestinal tract. She uses a powdered formula with a mixture of dried apricots to improve taste. She administers one-third teaspoon every morning before feeding Adam. She also gives Adam the cod liver oil, rich in vitamins A and D and essential unsaturated fatty acids. It's commonly referred to as the number one superfood. Heather reports, "My kids love it because I buy the kind that is flavored with lemon and orange which masks the fishy taste."

Heather's naturopath also recommended pulsatilla for Adam because he was becoming withdrawn socially. Pulsatilla is a remedy derived from the plant commonly known as wind flower and is native to central and northern Europe and southern England. This wild plant grows in sunny meadows, pastures, and fields. It is used to treat grief, anger, fright, shock, consumption of rich foods, and loss of vital fluids.

Over a year or so, Heather continued these homeopathic remedies and greatly reduced Adam's intake of dairy and wheat. She substituted cow's milk cheese with goat's milk cheese, as she was advised the molecules in goat's milk were smaller and easier to digest.

Some social situations are challenging and family dynamics are mixed for Heather. Because Heather's father-in-law is allergic to wheat, dairy and cane sugar, Heather says, "He and his wife are used to dealing with food allergies, so it is more comfortable when visiting. But other people, who are not used to the severity of today's food allergies in children, are not as experienced and it can be challenging to provide a safe food environment for my kids, especially when the allergens are not obvious, such as bread crumbs contained in meatballs or at birthday parties when I don't want Adam to feel excluded."

Heather admitted that, "For social reasons I have allowed Adam to eat birthday cake or other foods occasionally that contain cow's milk and wheat." Sometimes, babysitters would occasionally mistakenly give him these foods as well. She has found that even though there have been no hospital visits, his eczema has returned and his last naturopath visit and allergy test showed little improvement in his allergic reactions. Recently, she vowed to eliminate all amounts of cow's milk and wheat from his diet, regardless of social implications.

As for herself, during the last few years, Heather started developing some asthma. She was on vacation with her family when she started having a severe asthmatic attack. She thankfully used the inhaler she had but was scared by the severity of the attack. Her face and neck broke out in hives, while her eyes and fingers became swollen. Since learning that she is also allergic to dairy and wheat, she has avoided consuming these allergens. She happily reports, "Over the past two years I have been careful to avoid dairy and wheat, and my asthma is gone. I know that even the slightest bits of those foods affect me because when I used to put cream in my coffee, my eyes would puff up."

Heather will continue to feed herself and her family in accordance with her naturopath's instructions and will consume as many organic foods as possible. She is optimistic and is aware of the improved eating habits for her entire family that have come out of this difficult experience.

CHAPTER 13: KATHY'S STORY

Kathy is a thirty-one-year-old mother of two boys, one-and-a-half-year-old Brayden and three-and-a-half-year-old KC. She lives in the United States. Prior to having children she worked as a school counselor. Kathy's older son has no allergies whatsoever and eats a wide variety of foods. Brayden, her younger son, is allergic to dairy, eggs, peanuts, walnuts, dog hair and appears to have some seasonal allergies as well.

When Brayden was just one month old, he began to develop severe eczema, but Kathy didn't realize that it was eczema. She thought he just had sensitive skin. He was born in November and by December it was getting chilly and Kathy would wear her wool sweaters. Kathy says, "I thought the wool might be irritating his skin, especially since I was always holding him or breastfeeding him. So I stopped wearing the wool sweaters, but the eczema just got worse."

She brought Brayden to the pediatrician, who prescribed a cortisone cream and instructed Kathy to rub it all over Brayden's body. Kathy was not happy with this solution. "I wanted to know what was causing my son's eczema, not just treat the symptom," she says. So she asked the doctor if perhaps her son might have food allergies and should she start eliminating foods from her own diet. Her doctor *dis*agreed, stating that since only a small number of the foods she ate would enter her breast milk, it would not make a difference. So Kathy left the doctor's office, filled the prescription, but when she arrived at home, she felt, "this was just a band-aid solution to the symptom, not the real problem."

Kathy did not use the prescription cream. She tried over-the-counter moisturizing lotions and homeopathic recommendations, but unfortunately Brayden's eczema worsened. Kathy also tried to eliminate some foods from her own diet, but by the time he was three to four months, her baby was so uncomfortable that he could not sleep. Kathy recalls, "It was a nightmare. His eczema was so bad that he woke every fifteen minutes each night which continued for two weeks. I got no sleep. Neither did Brayden." Kathy called the pediatrician and explained that the situation had worsened. The pediatrician encouraged Kathy to try the cortisone cream again. This time Kathy took his advice, but did so reluctantly. She also tried giving Brayden some probiotics based upon the advice of her chiropractor.

These solutions helped but did not completely eliminate the eczema. She remembers, "I kept trying to find an answer. I went to the pharmacy and asked the pharmacist, an old friend of the family, for some advice. The pharmacist suggested some an over-the-counter cream that had been on the market for generations so it was "time-tested" as opposed to a newly invented concoction. I bought and tried this cream and it did seem to help. But I just wasn't satisfied that I was addressing the problem, only the symptom." Kathy's skepticism of her pediatrician was growing. Her husband was friendly with a naturopathic doctor who had some advice, but she wasn't sure she wanted to take this route either. Without any solution, Brayden and his mom continued to suffer with the severe eczema.

Brayden was now six months and Kathy began to introduce him to some solid foods. She found that he liked fruits and vegetables but did not care for oatmeal or rice. She was also breastfeeding while consuming dairy, eggs, peanuts and a wide variety of tree nuts in her own diet. Brayden still had eczema.

At nine months, Kathy tried to introduce dairy, by giving Brayden whole milk yogurt. Within a few minutes, he broke out in hives. Kathy explains, "I immediately called the pediatrician, but it took him forty-five minutes to call me back. By the time the doctor called, Brayden's hives had begun to go away. He told me to give him antihistamine if it happened again." Then two weeks later, Kathy tried giving Brayden some non-fat yogurt that was plain—had no other flavors or ingredients—but again the hives returned. This time she gave him antihistamine. She contacted the pediatrician who wanted her to conduct one more test by giving Brayden some plain cow's milk to confirm it was the milk and not the yogurt that was causing a reaction. When she tried again, Brayden's eyes began to swell, ooze and turn red. He also developed hives on his face. She recalls, "He looked like he had been in a fight."

Since Kathy was still breastfeeding, she now decided to eliminate all dairy, including all trace dairy found in breads, crackers, cookies as well as the obvious sources such as pizza and ice cream. She also eliminated eggs from her diet. Within a few weeks, she says, "Brayden's eczema cleared up by about ninety percent." Kathy was thrilled that she finally found the solution she'd been looking for over the past nine months. She did give him peanut butter at about fourteen months, because he wasn't eating any meat and only consumed a small amount of soy, so she thought he should have more protein. There was no negative reaction to the peanut butter.

Six months later, when Brayden was fifteen months, he underwent allergy and anemia testing by way of blood testing. Kathy learned he was "allergic to dairy (three on a scale of six), egg (two on a scale of six) and peanuts/tree nuts (one on a scale of six). He also tested positive for dog hair. The iron test showed no anemia." The pediatrician performed these tests then referred Kathy to an allergist. When she went to the allergist just one month ago, he felt that no additional tests were necessary. Kathy was interested in learning more about food allergies and the meaning of the results with respect to their severity. "But," she recalls, "I was disappointed with the amount of information that the allergist gave me. He didn't discuss allergies with me or the details of Brayden's reactions. I felt that the doctor hurried me out of the office with pamphlets and prescriptions for an EpiPen® Jr. and antihistamine."

Now that Brayden is eighteen months, he finally has found relief from eczema through careful food elimination. Kathy is thrilled, but continues to use non-prescription moisturizing creams on him to keep his skin moist and to see a naturopath for supplements. She finds it interesting that Brayden did not like the foods to which she has since found him to be allergic. "Perhaps our bodies know what is good for us and what is not," she wonders. "Now that I have some answers with respect to Brayden's health after searching for most of his life, I feel confident that following my instincts was the right thing to do," she says.

Having gone through this experience, she feels more compassion for other parents and children who suffer from food allergies. She recalls her days as a school counselor and believes that while empathy is important, keeping a positive attitude is equally important. She says, "I've tried to keep a positive attitude throughout this experience and I think I've been successful. Now that I am no longer breastfeeding, I can eat whatever I want which is a big relief and stress reducer. I am so thankful that my older son doesn't have any food allergies or problems trying new foods." This experience has taught Kathy to appreciate things she might otherwise not have appreciated.

CHAPTER 14: YAEL'S AND ORNIT'S STORY (ISRAEL)

Yael is a forty-eight-year-old mother of four who was born in Kfar Saba and grew up in Givatayim, Israel. Prior to having her fourth child, she worked for sixteen years in a traffic engineering office. She has been working as a full-time mother since her fourth was born. Her husband was born and grew up in Afula, Israel. Neither her family nor her husband's family has a known history of food allergies. Their four children range in age from nine to twenty years. Only Yael's youngest son, Noam, has food allergies.

When Noam was five months, Yael began to supplement his breast-fed diet with some infant formula because she felt he needed more to eat. Initially, she gave him a non-milk-based infant formula, but was soon encouraged by one of the nurses to change to a milk-based formula. Yael agreed to try the milk formula. After a few days on the milk-based formula, Yael recalls, "Noam had tiny little marks on his belly and his legs, which resembled mosquito bites. I remember that it puzzled me why these marks were on his belly. He used to sleep on his belly so perhaps that mattered I thought."

At the next doctor's visit, Yael mentioned the marks to the doctor. She also suggested that perhaps Noam was having an allergic reaction to the milk-based formula. She recalls, "The doctor did not think I was right." Yael took the doctor's advice and continued to supplement Noam's diet with milk-based formula. Shortly afterward, she noticed that the marks originally on his belly had spread to more of his body and to his head. Further, the marks were larger and Yael became scared. She brought Noam to the hospital where she explained that these marks only started to appear once she gave Noam milk-based formula. She asked the hospital personnel to give Noam an allergy test for milk, but they refused and told her that Noam simply had a virus.

When Yael brought Noam home from the hospital, he was tired and she felt exhausted. Again, she tried to believe the advice of the doctors at the hospital and reached for a bottle of the milk-based formula. She shook and fed it to Noam. Within seconds he vomited. Yael then knew that Noam was allergic to milk, regardless of what the doctors told her. She decided, at that point, to remove all milk from his diet and switched to a non-milk-based formula. She continued this diet for the remainder of his first year and the marks never reappeared.

Once Noam was over one year, Yael slowly began to introduce milk-based food products into his diet such as yogurt. Thankfully, there have been no further negative reactions. Noam is now nine years old and reported to her that, "[W]hen I drink milk-based cocoa or eat ice cream, it makes my throat ache." Yael always reminded Noam that he should avoid eating those foods. She noticed that Noam does not appear to have any reactions to yogurt or milk, but high protein dairy foods such as cheese will make him feel sick.

Yael recalls that when she decided that Noam was allergic to milk, "I felt very sorry for him. He wouldn't know the flavor of ice cream and many tasty things that are made from milk. Then I discovered all the products which are made of soy and other alternatives and I comforted myself that it wasn't that bad and would probably pass when he turned one year old." Noam's grandmother felt that his allergy was a disaster—especially in the beginning—but then she slowly came to accept the allergy and eventually no longer felt that way.

Now that Noam has mostly outgrown his allergy it no longer affects his family's life or his time at daycare. Yael found that the staff at the daycare was quite attentive to Noam's classmate who had a food allergy. Yael has noticed the increased incidence of children with food allergies in Israel in recent years. Awareness in society has grown as well. She recalls, "There was a time when my third child, Inbal, was in kindergarten and she asked me to bake a cake for her birthday that contains no eggs because one of her friends was allergic to eggs. I called the girl's mother and asked her for a recipe for such a cake. She gladly gave one to me and told me how appreciative she was."

Yael's husband's niece, Maytar, also suffers from food allergies. Maytar's mother, Ornit, is a thirty-eight-year-old mother of four, who was born and raised in Afula, Israel along with her husband. Neither has a known family history of food allergies. Prior to having her third child, Ornit worked for a transportation company as a secretary. Since her third, she is a full-time mother. Their children range from two to fourteen years. Only Ornit's third daughter, Maytar, has food allergies.

When Maytar was five months, Ornit began to add fruit and eggs to her diet. Soon after that, Maytar developed an itchy rash all over her body. Ornit took her to a dermatologist who prescribed a salve (ointment), but it was not effective. Quite frustrated, Ornit persisted and took her daughter to a specialist, who examined Maytar's skin on her forehead and diagnosed her with "atopic dermatitis," a symptom of food allergy. He instructed Ornit not to give Maytar certain foods, specifically, grapes, eggs, peanuts, tuna, some types of fish, purple food coloring (red and blue were okay) nor to allow her to touch sand or grass. The specialist said the only kind of fruits she should eat were banana, apple, pear and watermelon. Ornit was advised only to use specific shampoos, soaps and creams that would keep Maytar's skin moist and lubricated.

Maytar is now three years old and is aware of her own allergy most of the time. She even reminds adults to check what her food contains. Ornit recalls that when she found out about the allergy, "I was devastated. But, now we have learned to live with it." Ornit found, "The staff at the kindergarten was quite attentive to Maytar's food allergy. Even the parents of the other children, who were initially afraid their own children might catch the same condition, began to feel sorry for her. We even worked together to agree on a certain menu for birthday parties which will suit Maytar."

CHAPTER 15: CASSIE'S STORY

Cassie has a calm demeanor for her thirty-one years. She has one child, a son named Evan, who is two and one-half years old He is an adorable sturdy little blonde fellow who speaks quite well. She is also now four months pregnant with her second child. Prior to having children, she was an art teacher at a middle school, but now she is spending all of her time taking care of her home and child. She lives in the United States.

When Evan was six months, Cassie found blood in his diaper. Cassie brought him to the pediatrician's office and was told that Evan was too young to be tested for food allergies. He advised Cassie not to eat any dairy or soy as she was still breastfeeding and also not to give Evan any dairy or soy directly. The pediatrician said a dairy allergy wasn't life threatening and so did not prescribe an EpiPen® Jr. He advised that Evan would probably outgrow the allergy so Cassie should try giving him dairy every three months until no reaction appeared. The doctor seemed relaxed, which helped to calm her. Cassie was also helped by the fact that Evan was, "a laid back baby—he would spit up a lot, but would just giggle afterward, he was so calm," she remembers. Cassie followed the doctor's advice carefully and even postponed all solid foods for Evan until he was eight months.

About four months later, when Evan was one year, Cassie gave him a sippy-cup of milk. Right away Evan broke out in a bright red rash. Cassie called the pediatrician immediately and he advised her not to challenge Evan with dairy again. At this point he recommended that she take him to an allergist. Another important reaction occurred before the age of one as well. Cassie recalls a time when her husband was snacking on peanuts. He leaned over and kissed Evan. Within seconds a kissed-shaped welt appeared on Evan's face. Cassie knew at that point that Evan probably had an allergy to peanuts.

At the age of one, Cassie brought Evan to the allergist for the skin prick test. The results showed that he was allergic, as suspected, to dairy and peanut, but also to egg, which was unexpected. The allergist further recommended a blood test stating, "If a person was allergic to something in the past then the skin prick test will always show a positive result, even if they've since outgrown it."

The blood test also showed that Evan had outgrown the dairy allergy. But surprisingly, the allergist questioned whether Evan was really allergic to dairy. This seemed odd to Cassie since she saw Evan's reaction to milk, where he broke out in hives just a few weeks earlier. The allergist suggested that Cassie try milk with Evan again, but Cassie felt that it would be prudent to avoid milk for a bit longer.

The skin prick test results for the egg were surprising to Cassie as well. The results showed a moderate level of reaction to egg so the allergist advised her to avoid eggs. Cassie followed his advice and avoided egg, but would allow Evan to have egg if it was baked in a cake or bread since it was in small amounts and fully cooked. She has never seen Evan have any reaction to eggs. The allergist advised that even though she might not see a reaction, Evan might develop a stomachache.

When Evan was a bit over a year, Cassie introduced him to egg and he had no negative reactions. She waited for another year before giving him milk again at about two and one-half years. At that time, there was no negative reaction.

The allergist told Cassie never to feed peanuts to Evan or even allow him to be near them. She responded by eliminating peanuts from her house and making her own baked goods. She did not attempt to use any box cake mixes because they might contain traces of peanut. She is highly careful to avoid all foods that are manufactured in a facility that also manufactures products which contain peanuts. Eventually, after months of label checking she successfully found some prepared baked goods that did not contain peanuts at the local supermarket. She has given these foods to Even and because he has had no reactions whatsoever; the foods appear to be safe.

Cassie believes, "The peanut allergy is really scary because people tend to forget or are ignorant about food allergies, especially the highly sensitive peanut allergy. For example, I went to a party at my mother's and found a bowl of nuts on the table. I reminded my mom of Evan's peanut allergy and asked her to take the nuts away. My mom said she just hadn't thought of it. She apologized and put the nuts away."

On the other hand, Cassie feels her mother-in-law doesn't fully understand the extent of the allergy. Cassie says, "My mother-in-law will often ask if Evan can have just a little ice cream or pizza. I try to take a deep breath and remind her that Evan's allergy is serious and even a little bit is not good for him." Cassie thinks, "Times have changed since our mothers' generation. I think the older generations just don't always get it." Cassie and her husband understand and know of the seriousness of the peanut allergy from personal experience. Specifically, her husband knew a nineteen-year-old who died after having a few drinks at a bar along with a candy bar that contained peanuts.

Cassie's fear is enhanced because she feels peanuts are prevalent in our society as a snack food or part of snack foods. She explains, "There are so many things children eat that contain peanuts. Often Evan is nearby peanuts. I feel the best way to teach Evan to handle his allergy is to train him to understand that he has the allergy and to ask if the foods given to him might contain peanuts. For instance, when we go to restaurants I encourage Evan to ask the waitress if the foods contain peanuts. I want Evan to be his own advocate." When Evan starts preschool, Cassie wants to be sure the peanut allergy is well addressed. She plans on placing Evan in a drop off gymnastics class this fall where she feels the instructor is quite aware of his allergy and the snack time will be monitored closely.

Now that Cassie is expecting her second child, she is avoiding peanuts completely. She also stays away from dairy but will occasionally indulge in a bit of ice cream. Neither Cassie, nor her husband, has food allergies. They are not aware of any history of food allergies in their families.

Cassie's husband does have an immune system disorder which causes him a great deal of fatigue and he often gets welts and hives. He is currently on an asthma medication for this disorder even though he doesn't have asthma. The medication seems to work to calm his body of its reactions.

CHAPTER 16: STEPHANIE'S STORY

Stephanie is a forty-four-year-old mother of one daughter, Kim. Stephanie was a full-time English high school teacher prior to having a child and now teaches part-time at a university. She lives in the United States. Stephanie is contemplative as she seemed to consider questions and come back with more details a little while later during the interview—she likes to think about things.

Stephanie's daughter, Kim, is a pretty, petite girl of four years. Her mother described her as a bit shy, and I found her to be wholly pleasant, calming the playroom atmosphere with my two boys. Kim has been diagnosed as being allergic to dairy, eggs and peanuts but has since outgrown two of these allergies.

Before having her baby, Stephanie went to a lactation nurse to learn about breastfeeding. The nurse said to stay away from chocolate because it tends to bother babies since it contains a chemical that babies' digestive systems cannot handle. While breastfeeding Stephanie did occasionally indulge in chocolate, which she loves. She noticed that, indeed, Kim would be especially cranky after breastfeeding subsequent to eating chocolate. Stephanie recalls, "When I stopped eating chocolate, Kim's adverse reactions stopped." Stephanie drank and ate milk products while breastfeeding but did not notice any outward signs of negative effects on Kim. Stephanie also ate peanuts during her pregnancy and breastfeeding.

Stephanie noticed that Kim seemed to have gas during her first year, especially from about four months to seven months. It was especially apparent between the hours of eleven o'clock at night and two o'clock in the morning. She tried giving Kim an American-made medicine for gas but it didn't help. Then she learned about gripe water from her mother-in-law. Gripe water is a natural remedy for gas that her mother-in-law found in Ireland. Stephanie checked with the pediatrician, but he'd never heard of it. Stephanie tried it and found it worked well.

Stephanie continued to breastfeed Kim for a year. When Kim was one year, Stephanie tried to wean her by giving her some cow's milk. Immediately Kim's lip swelled and turned red. Her skin became blotchy, but she did not develop hives. Stephanie called the doctor who advised her that the allergy to milk is something children may or may not outgrow. He suggested trying soy milk, which Stephanie did with excellent results. She continued with the soy milk and breastfeeding until Kim was about fifteen months at which time she tried the cow's milk again, a few tablespoons at a time. She was pleased to see that there was no longer a reaction. At that time, Stephanie fully weaned Kim.

When Kim was about two years, Stephanie went to her sister's house. Her sister made Kim a poached egg. Stephanie cut it up into small pieces and gave a few bites to Kim. Within a few seconds, Kim's lip became red and swollen and the blotches appeared on her face. Stephanie immediately gave her some antihistamine and the reaction dissipated. Stephanie called the pediatrician, who advised her to try giving Kim the eggs again in about three months. Stephanie did try again, after three months, but Kim's reaction was the same: swollen red lips and blotchy skin. Three months later, when Kim was two and one-half years, Stephanie tried the eggs again and this time Kim showed no reaction.

"Also at about two and one-half years," Stephanie recalls, "a babysitter gave Kim a peanut butter cracker for the first time. Within fifteen minutes her face and lips swelled and the lips turned bright red. I was so frightened and called the pediatrician who recommended some antihistamine. Thankfully the reaction went away within ten to fifteen minutes. I made an appointment with the doctor for that afternoon. Since there was an allergist on staff at the pediatric office, he immediately sent Kim for an allergy test. After seven to ten days, the blood test confirmed that Kim was allergic to peanuts, but only mildly. No tree nut allergy was found. Since the peanut allergy was not severe, he didn't prescribe an EpiPen® Jr. and instead advised me to give Kim antihistamine if she had another reaction."

Stephanie felt that her doctor was good and she liked his calm demeanor. She tried to remain calm herself. She felt somewhat nervous though and asked herself, "What did I do wrong?" She says, "I want to always do the best as a parent." She went home with both some unanswered questions and new information about Kim's allergies.

For about a year, Stephanie was careful to avoid giving peanuts to Kim, but she continued to eat peanuts herself and allow the peanuts to be in the house. The day before Thanksgiving, when Kim was three and one-half years old, Stephanie went to her sister's house for the holiday. Stephanie remembers, "My sister and I were chatting and snacking on peanuts. I think I bent over and kissed Kim. Within ten to fifteen minutes, Kim had a huge lip." Stephanie described the size by pulling her own lip out at least an inch. Stephanie's sister called 911 and Stephanie gave Kim antihistamine immediately. In about ten minutes, the swelling started to go down and the paramedics arrived. The paramedics asked if Kim seemed to have trouble breathing or if she was coughing. Stephanie said, "No. But what should we do now?"

The paramedics advised Stephanie that the reaction seemed to be from the peanut allergy. They explained that Stephanie had several options depending upon how she wanted to handle the situation. She could have them bring Kim to the hospital for treatment. Or she could keep Kim at home and watch her for another possible reaction later in the evening. If another reaction occurred, she'd need to call the paramedics again. They explained that the next reaction could cause her to stop breathing and could happen in the middle of the night. Stephanie was distraught. She says, "I was frustrated since I didn't know what to do and no one was giving me a recommendation, only options." Although she felt unsure about what to do, she felt the safest route was to have the paramedics take Kim to the hospital for treatment right then. She also realized that she would probably need an EpiPen® should a reaction occur again."

So about ten minutes after the paramedics arrived, Stephanie boarded the ambulance with her daughter. Once at the hospital, she advised them of Kim's weight, about twenty-six pounds. They administered a liquid steroid to Kim to help prevent any breathing distress. Stephanie advised the staff that Kim was pre-asthmatic, since she had had two asthmatic episodes. (Three episodes are required to be defined as asthmatic.) Eventually the swelling completely subsided and the hospital released Kim giving her two prescriptions: one for an EpiPen® and one for antihistamine.

By that time it was ten o'clock at night and Stephanie was exhausted from the emotions she had felt throughout the day. She went to the pharmacy to get the prescription filled since the following day was Thanksgiving and she thought the drug stores would not be open. At the pharmacy, the young woman pharmacist assistant looked at the prescription for the EpiPen® and told Stephanie, "This is the wrong dosage. You need the green box (EpiPen® Jr.) not the yellow box which is for an adult." Stephanie looked back at her in disbelief. She wasn't sure if the hospital had made a mistake or if this young pharmacist was overstepping her bounds.

Stephanie felt the prudent thing to do was to double check the prescription, so the pharmacist assistant called the hospital. She reported to Stephanie that the doctor was standing by his original dosage. The pharmacist assistant reluctantly filled the prescription and Stephanie went back to her sister's house for the Thanksgiving holiday. Stephanie recalls, "I was so tired and upset."

The Friday following Thanksgiving Stephanie took Kim to the pediatrician. The nurse looked at the box of the EpiPen® and immediately said it was the wrong dosage—it was for an adult, not a child. The pediatrician confirmed this. Stephanie was internally irate but tried to remain outwardly calm. She discussed the entire event with the pediatrician. She says, "Not only did the hospital give the wrong dosage, but they failed to train me how to use the EpiPen®!" Another blood test was taken. After seven to ten days the results confirmed that the level was mild but that Stephanie should have an EpiPen® Jr. on hand. Stephanie asked the doctor what might have happened to Kim if she received the adult dosage EpiPen®. The doctor said Kim probably would have been all right just very hyperactive for awhile. Stephanie also discussed this with a friend of hers who said, "My allergist told me that an adult EpiPen® could cause heart failure in a child because of the amount of adrenaline." Stephanie decided to follow up with the hospital about the mistake that the doctor had made.

She called the hospital three times over the span of ten days before she received a response. The director of the hospital was in transition so a liaison called her back and admitted that the EpiPen® dosage that had been prescribed was incorrect. Stephanie recalls, "He frantically asked me if I had used that EpiPen® on Kim. He then took a deep breath, a sort of sigh of relief, when she responded that she had not. I asked him, 'Why are you asking? What would have happened?' But he did not give me an answer. He was vague and said he just wanted to know."

Stephanie remained adamant with the hospital. She says, "I wanted three things: (1) an apology; (2) some assurance that it would not happen again to another child; and (3) reimbursement for the original incorrect EpiPen® for which she had to pay." To this date, almost a year later, she reports, "I have only received an apology. No assurance or letter has ever been given to me that the doctor who made the mistake would be reprimanded. No reimbursement has been given to me for the EpiPen® that I can't use."

So although Stephanie originally tried to handle her daughter's food allergies in a calm way and not to overreact, this experience has made her into a much more cautious parent. Because of this difficult experience and the allergist's recommendation, Stephanie decided to remove all peanuts from her home and Kim's environment. Stephanie now double checks all ingredients and carries a survival pack wherever she goes. Her pack includes antihistamine, the EpiPen® Jr. and an asthma inhaler. She takes a deep breath and says, "I tried to remain calm but I am not a happy camper when people make mistakes like what happened that horrible day at the hospital."

Stephanie has been advised by the allergist that Kim might outgrow the allergy by age five. Stephanie wants people to know, "Food allergy reactions occur without intention. People don't intentionally try to give kids food they're allergic to. It just happens. Furthermore, I find the older generation can be defensive, opinionated and unsupportive. It seems the grandparent generation doesn't want to ask questions and simply doesn't understand the extent of today's food allergy reactions."

She researched why the allergies to peanuts are so much more common today than they were when she was a child. She learned that peanuts used to be fried and now they are dry roasted. The frying process would remove the impurities in the peanuts, but the dry roasting does not. Therefore, the chemicals and pesticides remain in the peanuts and help to cause an allergic reaction.

Stephanie also feels chemicals affect her own body. She suffers from lactose intolerance and IBS (irritable bowel syndrome). Interestingly, when she travels outside of the United States and consumes dairy, her symptoms magically disappear. She has also noticed that "free range" is big in other countries and perhaps the naturalness of the foods there might agree with her digestive system better. Her experiences have led her to believe that the chemicals used and the food processing in the United States might be the cause of her digestive problems.

CHAPTER 17: DIANE'S STORY (NEW ZEALAND)

Diane is a forty-something mother of three boys. She was born in London and was raised in England and then New Zealand. Her husband was born in Invercargill, New Zealand where they now live. Prior to having children, Diane was an office manager and now works as a self-employed property administrator. Their three boys, ages nine, seven and four, are all allergic to dairy, egg, tree nuts, penicillin and dust mites.

The eldest son, Jonathon, was less than six months when Diane noticed his skin was itchy and red. She did not know that the skin condition was caused by food allergies. She brought Jon to the doctor who prescribed some creams and mild steroids. He also recommended giving Jon an antihistamine. Diane followed the doctor's advice but otherwise did not know what was wrong with her son. She recalls, "I often felt tired, frustrated and helpless."

When Jon was not quite a year, she tried giving him milk. He broke out in hives immediately. Diane gave him an antihistamine, which calmed his symptoms. The same reaction occurred when Jon was fourteen months and she tried feeding him some egg. Diane gave him more antihistamine. Then again, when Jon was about two years, Diane recalls, "One morning he helped himself to some muesli cereal for breakfast that contained nuts. Jon started making an awful noise as he tried to breathe. His throat was closing. I reached my fingers into his mouth and pulled out the nut and cereal. I immediately gave him more antihistamine and thankfully the reaction subsided quickly."

This type of minor accidental exposure occurred several times during Jon's nine years. Each time, Diane gave him an antihistamine but saw no point in calling the doctor. While she felt a certain level of helplessness, she began to feel like she was in more control since the antihistamine worked well. She took Jon to see an allergist to verify to what he was allergic. He was given both the skin prick and blood tests. The results showed that he was severely allergic to dairy, eggs and tree nuts. The results were the same for all three of her boys. Diane says, "To make matters worse, Jon has developed alopecia, complete hair loss. No one is sure whether the alopecia is caused by or related to the food allergies, although it is believed to be related to stress."

When Diane and her husband considered their family histories and food allergies, they found that both sides had a history of both eczema and asthma. She explains, "My husband is allergic to cracked pepper and his aunty has a nut allergy—her throat gets itchy when she eats nuts." Diane has support from friends and relatives, but also believes, "Like anything unless you've experienced something yourself, it can be quite difficult to understand what we go through everyday. It's not a cold or flu. It doesn't go away, unfortunately." She feels, "My relatives are sympathetic but really have no idea how difficult it can be." Sometimes, people will say to Diane, "I don't know if I could handle my child having allergies and eczema." Diane has to wonder if they hear what they are saying as she finds it rather insensitive. On a positive note, some friends, especially around birthday parties, have been extremely helpful and reassuring with appropriate party food. Furthermore, the daycare that Diane uses is very supportive and does not allow certain foods to be included in the other children's lunchboxes, such as tree nuts, kiwi fruits and fish, although they do allow dairy, egg and wheat.

Diane describes how frustrating it can be to have not just one, but three, children with food allergies. She stated, "The problem is more around what foods off the supermarket shelf they can and cannot have. I read and re-read labels all the time, every visit. It adds an enormous amount of time to food shop for my family. Another frustration is the inability to be spontaneous and eat anywhere or with anyone, whether it's a lunch or dinner out, or even enjoy the holidays in other countries." As Diane persists in feeding her children allergen-free foods, she is encouraged and says, "My boys are unlikely to have weight issues since they don't load up on cheesy pizzas and chocolate biscuits." Over time, Diane as also found, "There are more and more foods available for allergic people and even this week I have discovered more products that I am able to purchase for the boys."

Diane keeps a positive attitude and believes, "It is important to keep the child's spirit strong. Each child has to be incredibly disciplined and alert. I don't like him to think he is special because he can't have certain foods. I just keep my explanations simple by saying that some foods will make him very sick or possibly die. But my children are not missing out on much in the scheme of life. There's more to life than dairy, egg and nuts. Life only gives you what you can handle! I live in hope, keep faith and thank my lucky stars that it is just food allergies and not something far more sinister. If I could change it and make the allergies go away, of course, I would. But these are the cards that we've been dealt. I consider my three boys and husband the four aces! I'm a lucky mother and wife."

CHAPTER 18: MICHELLE'S STORY

Michelle is a thirty-five-year-old mother of two with plans to have a third child. Both she and her husband, Joe, were born in New York. Michelle has continued to work outside of the home as a management consultant and is now an associate controller for a prominent private university. Only Andy, Michelle's first born, suffers from food allergies. He is now five. His little sister, Mae, is three and allergy-free. Neither Joe nor Michelle has a known history of food allergies in his or her family.

When Andy was born, Michelle and Joe sensed something was wrong. "I nursed Andy for three weeks, but it did not go well. He always seemed cranky and hungry. We switched to formula, but then he vomited and had blood in his stools. He also cried constantly." Michelle tried different formulas made from soy but with no luck. She then tried the pre-digested, expensive brand of formula and Andy was like a different baby. He stopped crying and became a happy baby. When she reported these findings to Andy's doctor, he advised her that Andy had a dairy intolerance but was not truly allergic to dairy.

When Andy was nine months, Michelle started to feed him small pieces of table food. She gave him some macaroni and cheese. Within seconds he broke out in hives, and his tongue and eyes swelled. Michelle knew that he was having an allergic reaction. She called the doctor who advised her to give Andy some antihistamine and bring him into the office. She recalls the experience, "It was terrifying. I rode in the back of the car with him the whole way scared his throat would close up. I felt an array of mixed emotions. I was scared that he could go into anaphylactic shock."

She remembers, "I felt so angry with the doctor and myself for listening to him—he said Andy wasn't truly allergic to dairy. In my heart, I knew that Andy had a severe problem with dairy. My anger with the doctor was made worse because I felt that *he thought* I was overreacting." Now she knew that she should have trusted her own intuition and insight more than the doctor's advice. She vowed never to make that mistake again, stating, "From that moment on I took charge of my son's allergies."

With newly found confidence, she took Andy to an allergist and had him tested. Both the skin prick and blood test were performed. When Andy was nine months his results showed that his reactions were very high for both dairy and eggs. His blood test results were twenty-five for dairy (on a scale of one to fifteen), and five for egg (on a scale of one to five). Michelle was surprised to learn about the egg allergy because Andy had never eaten eggs. But she accepted it because when he came into contact with egg through cross-contamination or physical contact with someone who had eaten eggs, he would break out in hives and begin to swell.

When Michelle and Joe realized the severity of Andy's food allergies, they decided the best thing for him would be to keep him at home until kindergarten or at least as long as possible. Joe stayed at home with the children for the first three and one-half years of Andy's life. Joe baked bread at home and kept both children on a dairy and egg-free diet, even though only Andy suffers from food allergies. Both were kept on the same diet because when Mae was one year, Michelle and Joe allowed her to have a bottle of cow's milk but found that it would splash on the floor or otherwise come into contact with Andy causing him to break out in hives. Based on that experience and the doctor's advice, they've found it easier to keep Mae on the same diet as Andy, at least until they are older.

Before Joe headed back to work, they toured many daycare centers. It was difficult because the staffs could not provide the safe food environment that Michelle and Joe wanted. Michelle recalls, "We were terrified by the lack of knowledge and systems in place for dealing with food allergies. They did not make me feel confident that Andy would not ingest dairy or eggs. One daycare provider told us flat out that she could not guarantee that the children would wash their hands after eating a snack that contained dairy or egg so that Andy would not break out in hives. We were dumbfounded." Furthermore, most daycare personnel said that their son would be seated at a table by himself for all meals. It made Michelle and Joe feel terribly sad to picture Andy eating alone.

Although all the daycare centers visited were peanut-free it provided no relief for Michelle and Joe's situation because Andy wasn't allergic to peanuts, but rather egg and dairy. Michelle and Joe finally decided to select a daycare whose kitchen wall and food carts displayed which children were allergic to which foods. Furthermore, the teachers were trained in food allergies and a teacher would be designated to sit next to each allergic child during all meals. Michelle liked the fact that Andy did not have to sit by himself, but he could sit with the other children, under the supervision of the teacher. Even better, the cook had experience in cooking for children with food allergies.

During the past eighteen months, there have been two food related incidents at the daycare. First, when Andy was eating lunch, he grabbed a cup of cow's milk from the table and accidentally drank it. He realized it tasted different and took another sip to check it again. Then, he picked up his soy milk cup and took a sip of that to see if it was the right cup. Then, the teacher saw him with two cups in his hand and panicked. She asked Andy if he drank the milk. He responded, "No." Then she asked again, "Andy, you need to tell me! Did you drink milk? This time, he said, "Yes." The teacher did not know which answer to believe.

Unfortunately, the teacher hoped for the best and did nothing. Within a short time, Andy began vomiting and coughing from the mucus he developed. Michelle and Joe were on their way from work and gave Andy some antihistamine immediately. Michelle recalls, "We explained to the daycare center that regardless of whether Andy drank the milk, he should have been given the antihistamine because there was a chance that he had drunk the milk." Andy's symptoms continued in the form of breathing problems and diarrhea for days. Michelle administered his breathing treatments as needed. Although Michelle recalls this rather nightmarish experience with frustration, she points out the positive aspect was that Andy did not go into anaphylactic shock.

The second incident at the daycare was when Andy accidentally ate bread and butter made with cow's milk butter rather than his normal dairy-free "butter." The daycare center did not tell Michelle and Joe what happened until the end of the day when they picked him up. Michelle recalls, "Joe and I were furious!" Andy did not have a reaction, but he had a stomachache that night at home. A lesson learned for the daycare included having a better plan for serving food and responding to incidents in which a child may have ingested an allergy producing food.

Now that Andy is five, he remains highly allergic to dairy, a ten (on a scale of one to fifteen), but he appears to have outgrown his allergy to eggs, for which he will soon be given a challenge test. His dairy reactions continue to produce hives, vomiting, diarrhea and mucus in the lungs. Michelle is told that Andy has "reactive airways," an asthma symptom and requires prescription breathing treatments for days to treat it.

Michelle remembers, "Andy's food allergies were terrifying for so many years but now are manageable. We bring Andy-friendly-food wherever we go. Recently we have gone to restaurants where we can specifically tell the cook how to prepare and Andy-friendly-meal." The hardest part of Andy's food allergies is that Michelle and Joe feel badly that Andy cannot eat what all the other kids can eat. He always has his own homemade cupcake at parties, but he cannot eat pizza or other dairy treats. Andy is now just starting to say, "It isn't fair!" Michelle agrees with him but tries to remind him of all the great things he can eat and that one day he will be able to eat pizza.

Another hard part about dealing with the food allergies involves family and relatives. Michelle stated, "My relatives do not take it seriously enough. One time, my mother-in-law did not think it was a big deal to stir her dairy mashed potatoes and then use the same spoon to stir Andy's soy mashed potatoes. They all thought we were overreacting until Andy would break out in hives or vomit from a meal. For years, we would not let anyone watch our children and we would never let them eat anyone else's food. Now our families have a clearer understanding, but even this past weekend my mother-in-law used the same spoon to serve herself something with dairy and then give Andy a scoop of peas. We caught it just in time and cleared the peas off Andy's plate. She said she was sorry and that she just wasn't thinking." Friends are a lot easier. Michelle believes their friends are very supportive and ask a lot of questions. She says, "They know I will always ask what they are serving so that I can bring an Andy-friendly alternative. Some of them even go out of their way to serve Andy-friendly-food."

Another positive note is that Michelle feels that she and Joe are better parents for having to deal with severe food allergies. Michelle proudly reports, "Our children have never eaten fast food. They don't even know what a donut is. I think if we were not managing this food allergy, we would not be eating as healthy as we are. Ever since my children were young, they always loved eating fruits for dessert. Now they can also have dairy-free, egg-free Oreos and soy ice cream."

A final piece of advice that Michelle would like to share is that she has created a "babysitter spreadsheet" that they hang on their refrigerator. The babysitter spreadsheet explains the children's schedule, doctor's emergency phone numbers, medication instructions, and what Andy can and cannot eat. Michelle says, "Our mantra to friends, family, and babysitters is: When in doubt leave it out...Don't give it to Andy." They also have a printed copy of, "How to read a label for egg and dairy ingredients."

Furthermore, their foods are labeled with red X's on boxes that are not Andy-friendly, and they label leftover containers in the refrigerator similarly. Michelle explains, "Whenever anyone watches our children now, which is limited to a select few, we go over all written instructions with them. Once we left our children with Joe's parents for four days. I gave them emergency medical treatment forms for each child that included Andy's allergic reactions, oral medications, inhaled medications, his medical treatment plan from his asthma and allergy specialist, and our insurance card. Everything went smoothly, thankfully."

CHAPTER 19: CATHERINE'S STORY

Catherine is a forty-eight-year-old mother of two grown children and works as a freelance photographer. Her son, who is twenty-seven, has no food allergies but her daughter, who is nineteen, was diagnosed with celiac disease in high school.

When Catherine's daughter, Amy, was a baby, she did not exhibit any food allergy symptoms, but she was colicky. Catherine remembers, "Amy was very gassy as a baby. I could feel her tummy rumbling from the bubbles in her abdomen. I tried anti-gas medication, but it didn't help too much." When Amy was about eleven, she began to complain of stomachaches. She also complained of aches and pains in her joints. Catherine said she took Amy to the doctor, who x-rayed her, but found nothing and said she was fine. Two years later, when Amy was thirteen, Catherine took her to an endocrinologist and suggested that Amy might have issues relating to food. The doctor ran some tests and reported that there were no issues and perhaps Amy had IBS, Irritable Bowel Syndrome (a spastic colon is a functional bowel disorder characterized by abdominal pain and changes in bowel[15]).

Then when Amy was in her last year at high school, age seventeen, she lost twenty-five pounds. Amy was not on a diet and was eating the same amounts that she normally ate. She was an average size prior to losing the weight but was quite thin after the loss. Catherine remembers, "She constantly complained of diarrhea, acid reflux in her throat, and aches and pains in her joints. She was out of school for seventeen days that school year and was at risk for not graduating due to too many absences. Then, one morning I was listening to the radio and heard a woman explain the symptoms of celiac disease. I was stunned. The description was exactly what Amy was suffering."

Catherine again brought Amy back to the doctor and insisted that she be tested for celiac disease. Again the doctor said that Amy was probably suffering from IBS. Then Catherine explained what she had heard on the radio and again asked the doctor to test Amy for celiac disease. The doctor finally agreed, saying that the test was a simple blood test. Indeed, Catherine was correct, Amy had celiac disease.

Celiac disease is caused by an intolerance to gluten (not an allergy), a substance found in wheat, rye and barley grains. The disease causes the villi in the small intestine, the tiny fingerlike protrusions lining the small intestine, to be damaged or destroyed. Since the villi normally allow nutrients from food to be absorbed into the bloodstream, without them, a person becomes malnourished regardless of the quantity of food eaten. Celiac disease is extremely difficult to diagnose without a blood test, especially in young children. The most common symptoms in young children are irritability, distended stomach, stunted growth, mild anemia, diarrhea and constipation.

The doctor then suggested that Amy see a gastroenterologist to confirm the diagnosis further. When Catherine took Amy, as recommended, the doctor wanted Amy to have an endoscopic biopsy of her small intestines to determine the extent of the damage. The procedure was done along with a colonoscopy. The results showed that Amy also had colitis. The doctor advised Amy that there is no cure for celiac disease, but a lifelong commitment to a gluten-free diet was imperative to treat the disease.

Within six months on the gluten-free diet, Amy's colon had healed itself and her acid reflux had stopped. Furthermore, she had gained back the twenty-five pounds even though she did not eat any additional amounts of food. Unlike before, her body was now absorbing all of the nutrients from the foods that she ate. In fact, the change by eliminating gluten was so dramatic that ten pounds was gained back in one month alone. Catherine remembers, "It was a wonderful thing to know that after six years of searching, we had finally found an answer for Amy."

Now Amy is in her sophomore year in college and is struggling with the social aspects of maintaining a gluten-free diet. She often feels isolated mostly because so much of college social life revolves around eating. Catherine says, "At first Amy's friends could not understand why she was not able to have just one piece of pizza. However, now that they are more informed about the disease they've become supportive and understanding." Going to restaurants, the cafeteria and people's houses for dinner is not easy. For instance, at restaurants and cafeterias, the frying oil used to cook gluten-containing foods can contaminate a gluten-free food. Furthermore, a salad might be contaminated by a crouton touching the salad.

Catherine is trying to educate Amy's college cafeteria staff about gluten and has asked the chef to make some gluten-free foods so that Amy can enjoy a meal with her friends rather than eating alone in her dorm room day after day. Currently, the gluten-free food that Amy can eat is not as easily accessible as Catherine and Amy would like. Further the choices of gluten-free foods are quite limited. The lack of progress, over the past year or so, has been frustrating for both of them. Catherine has done a great deal of research and tried to educate students and staff at Amy's college—even setting up a presentation on campus on celiac disease. Catherine reports, "Even a tiny amount of gluten, such as the size of one's pinky fingernail, can be enough to send the small intestine into shutdown mode." Therefore, Amy must not eat any gluten at all to avoid the consequences of celiac disease.

One of the many consequences of celiac disease is infertility. Amy plans on having children someday and is highly motivated to stay on her gluten-free diet for this reason. Celiac disease is an autoimmune disease and can, therefore, trigger other autoimmune diseases such as lupus and cancer. Other illnesses that are caused by celiac disease include malnutrition, anemia, and osteoporosis. Miscarriage and congenital malformation, such as neural tube defects, are risks for the baby of pregnant women who unknowingly suffer from celiac disease and continue to eat a diet containing gluten. The fetus doesn't get the nutrients it needs from the mother's body.

Catherine began to wonder how Amy got celiac disease since no one in their family has the disease. She and her husband had blood tests and found that her husband carries the gene for celiac disease. She also learned that in order to trigger the disease into action, a person usually undergoes a traumatic event such as pregnancy or an illness. Catherine recalls, "Amy had Roto virus when she was four and Lyme disease when she was eleven. Perhaps one of those illnesses weakened her body so it succumbed to the celiac disease that lay dormant in her body. Amy was always slightly anemic and tired—perhaps she never could fully absorb the iron from her foods that her body required."

Catherine's mission is to inform others of this disease, so that they might become aware of its symptoms and consequences. Catherine advises, "Don't stop searching for answers for your child if you believe something is wrong. Even if the doctors aren't listening to you, try another doctor and insist on the tests that you think will identify your child's illness. It might not be that the doctor's lack of help is intentional. It might just be that he or she doesn't normally test for celiac disease or isn't considering it. Don't give up—read, research and talk to others."

Michelle is a kind thirty-five-year-old mother of two boys ages four and five and one-half. She lives in the United States. Prior to becoming a stay-at-home mother, she was a medical marketing communications specialist. Now she cares for two very different boys, each with his own needs.

Harrison is Michelle's older son, who will be six soon. Four years ago, it was Easter morning and he ate a candy from his Easter basket that contained hazelnuts. Within minutes he vomited and developed hives all over his entire body. Michelle immediately gave him antihistamine and the hives disappeared within twenty minutes. He then developed diarrhea a bit later. Michelle thought the candy made him sick, but did not guess that he might be allergic to the hazelnut in the candy.

About three months later when the whole family was at a party at the home of Michelle's sister-in-law, the same scene occurred again when Harrison ate a homemade cookie that was decorated with a chocolate Rollo candy and a pecan squashed in the center. Harrison immediately vomited, developed hives and later had diarrhea. Michelle again gave him antihistamine, which calmed his symptoms successfully.

About six months later at a play date the hostess put out a plate of cookies. Harrison gleefully grabbed a walnut cookie and took a bite. Within seconds he vomited. It was then that Michelle put the three incidences together to connect the common thread of nuts in all of these foods, causing Harrison to react so adversely. Harrison was almost three now and Michelle brought him to an allergist for testing. She learned that he is highly allergic to tree nuts, showing a blood test sensitivity of five (on a scale of one to six).

Michelle says, "I am terrified that Harrison could have died from eating the foods with nuts in them during his second year of life. I also feel bad that I did not call the doctor after the first or second incident, or link the reactions to nuts until after the third one." After carefully avoiding tree nuts for two years, Michelle took Harrison to a naturopath for some additional allergy testing. The naturopath confirmed that Harrison has a true allergy to tree nuts and could go into anaphylactic shock if he consumed any. She also learned that Harrison has sensitivities, not allergies, to wheat and dairy. For his overall health, she now avoids these foods in his diet.

Michelle's second son, Mitchell is almost four. When he was about fifteen months, Michelle began to feel that Mitchell might not be meeting his developmental milestones as readily as other children do. Specifically, he was not yet walking and his verbal skills were not good. She decided to take some action and called an agency named "Birth to Three" to help her son. The counselor came to Michelle's home once a week for about a year to evaluate and work with Mitchell to help him develop. But she did not diagnose Mitchell with any developmental disorders, which gave Michelle some relief.

Although there was no diagnosis from the agency, Michelle still had a nagging feeling that Mitchell's behavior was not as it should be. Based on his verbal skills and aggressive behavior, Michelle explains, "I began to investigate and research these clues using the Internet and reading books. I found a test on the Internet for autism. Once all of the questions were answered, the score I was given for Mitchell showed he had a seventy percent positive diagnosis of PDDNOS (Pervasive Development Disorder Not Otherwise Specified)—which means a child has marked impairment of social interaction, communication, and/or behavior patterns."

She then decided to bring Mitchell to a neurologist shortly after his third birthday. The neurologist confirmed her findings about PDDNOS. Mitchell had been in preschool for about three months by this time. Michelle says, "I began to ask myself, and others, what can I do help Mitchell?"

The preschool advised Michelle that Mitchell wasn't really getting the benefits of preschool because his behavioral issues could not be addressed sufficiently by the teachers. Michelle asked the preschool teachers if they could communicate these issues to her school district for additional help. Unfortunately, because the preschool was in a different district from Mitchell's home town school district, they could not do that. Instead they recommended that she move Mitchell to a preschool in the same town as their residence. She complied and signed him up for the next semester at a more local preschool.

About the same time, a friend gave Michelle a book called Autism PDD written by a mother of an autistic child. Michelle remembers, "I learned that this mother eliminated wheat and gluten from her son's diet to help cure her son's autism. I decided to follow suit and also to have Mitchell tested by a naturopath. The test results showed that Mitchell was sensitive to gluten and dairy, so I eliminated both of these foods from his diet in addition to high fructose corn syrup." She also gave Mitchell vitamin and other supplements recommended by the naturopath most importantly DMG (Dimethylglycine), as well as fish oil, a multivitamin and calcium/magnesium, which he still has trouble taking because he doesn't like the taste.

There was about one month left in the current semester. During this time, Michelle made these dietary changes. Mitchell then started his new school. Within one week of starting (a total of five weeks on the new diet), Michelle had a thrilling moment. She explains, "I was holding Mitchell one day after school and he looked up at me and said, 'Mom, I colored today at school.' It was his first full sentence after years of practically no verbal communication! It was a clear sentence, not just a cryptic word or two strung together. I was stunned and couldn't believe it. I was thrilled!"

Michelle vows to continue this new diet in the hope that it will also help Mitchell's aggressive behavior issues as well. Specifically, she finds that he is not as aware of other children's feelings as she might like. She believes most little boys are somewhat physical, but his desire to wrestle, push and tackle other children is not the norm.

He has now been on this restricted diet for about six months. Michelle is still pleased with the verbal improvements but continues to work on the physical issues. She also has Mitchell in Occupational Therapy, which recommends brushing Mitchell's arms and legs two times a day to help calm his energies and finding an activity for Mitchell that helps to release his energy when he shows aggressive behavior.

Overall, Michelle says, "I am astonished at the chemicals in the popular big manufacturer foods—it is junk." She watches the commercials on TV and comments on the poor quality of these foods pushed so hard onto our children. She will continue keeping her first son's diet tree nut-free and her second son's diet dairy, gluten and high fructose corn syrup-free. Interestingly, she's found that many gluten-free foods tend to be made from a tree nut base. This makes it complicated and difficult for Michelle when trying to find foods that her whole family can eat.

To further add to the confusion, Michelle's husband was recently advised that he has sensitivity to wheat. The burden on Michelle to feed her family an allergen-free meal is stressful. She continues to try to serve more fruits and vegetables since they are allergen-free, but her children aren't used to consuming these natural foods.

Michelle states, "I'm becoming less and less happy with our pediatrician. He doesn't listen to me and I feel he doesn't know my son. I like the naturopath and am going to use that doctor more and carefully continue to select healthy, allergen-free foods for my family."

CHAPTER 21: KATIE'S STORY WITH ADHD

Katie is a vivacious and bright thirty-seven-year-old mother of three children. Prior to having children, she was a chemist. Recently earning her Masters in secondary education, she is now teaching high school chemistry. Neither she nor her husband has a known history of food allergies. None of her children exhibited true allergic reactions to food when they were babies or older. Only the middle child, Simon, exhibited some food sensitivities as a baby. He appeared to have a great deal of gas after consuming dairy and cried a lot.

When Simon was four, he entered preschool. Katie explains, "Both Simon's preschool teacher and I started noticing that Simon's behavior was not like most of the other children. He was extremely fidgety, was constantly on the move, and had trouble waiting in lines. He couldn't seem to wait for his turn to speak or keep his hands to himself when around his classmates. He also had a habit of getting too close to people when speaking with them." Katie felt Simon also appeared to be excessively anxious at times. Because Simon was only four and was a boy, Katie and the teacher decided to work with him in hope that Simon would change by the time he reached kindergarten. They both knew that he would be required to sit still to learn how to read in kindergarten. This was something that was impossible for Simon to do.

In the spring when Simon was five, Katie took him to his kindergarten screening. During the screening the kindergarten teacher watched Simon closely. Katie recalls, "When Simon was nervous, his behavior became worse. Since he was nervous during this kindergarten screening, it was easy to observe the hyperactive behavior." After the screening process, the kindergarten teacher contacted his preschool teacher to inquire as to whether his hyperactive behavior appeared in preschool as well. The preschool teacher reported that unfortunately he did indeed exhibit hyperactive behavior.

Katie also remembers that Simon's behavior appeared to be cyclical. Sometimes it was much worse than others. She remembers, "Simon's sleep routine was not good. I would put him to bed around seven o'clock, but he would be unable to fall asleep until eleven o'clock. Then he would often wake during the night. The disruptive sleep pattern would make him even more tired, which made it more difficult for him to fall asleep again the next night—it would set up a bad cycle." Based upon these observations, Katie and her husband, Keith, decided to take Simon to a neurologist.

Katie found a neurologist who specialized in pediatrics and ADHD. She and Keith brought Simon to this doctor. While they were all in the office together, the doctor began to discuss Simon's behavior. Katie and Keith grew increasingly uncomfortable as the doctor spoke. She says, "We could see that Simon was listening to what the doctor was saying about him. We began to worry that Simon's feelings and self-esteem might be hurt." Then the doctor gave them ADHD evaluations for the teacher and them to fill out describing Simon's daily behavior. After these tests were reviewed, Simon was labeled with ADHD, specifically with hyperactive tendencies. At this point the neurologist prescribed the drug Focalin XR (a form of Ritalin).

Upon returning home, Katie gave the Focalin XR to Simon and continued to do so for the next eight days. "His behavior changed," Katie recalls, "It became worse. Simon grew angry and violent. He began to say terrible things such as, 'I hate you' to me and he was hitting. Then Simon's kindergarten teacher called me to ask why he might be acting with an unusual and negative behavior." Katie and Keith could not take the behavior any longer so they called the neurologist. The doctor said Simon should stop taking the Ritalin. He asked them to come back to the office, where he wanted to do a brain scan on Simon to rule out a brain tumor. Katie and Keith watched Simon undergo an EEG. The doctor found no physical problems with Simon's brain pattern. He then suggested that Simon try yet another medication from the antidepressant family. At this point, Katie and Keith were not impressed with the neurologist's methods and said, "No, we don't want to place Simon on an antidepressant." They left and did not return.

Simon suffered in kindergarten and struggled with his social skills and academics. He had a great deal of trouble sitting still and could not learn to read because of it. His friendships suffered because he had difficulty listening to others, not touching them and not getting too close to them. He tended to participate in team sports late in a game and had a hard time stopping when the game was over. He was friends with girls more than boys, as the boys seemed less tolerant of his behavior. In the middle of the school year, Simon turned six and Katie began to wonder what else could be done to help him.

Katie recalls, "I began to call my friends to ask for some advice. One friend's son was autistic and another friend's son had food allergies. Both boys seemed to improve through a diet of food elimination. Both friends recommended the same naturopath doctor. So I took Simon to see the same doctor, who also happened to specialize in ADHD. Apparently he gives speeches throughout the country at naturopath doctor conferences."

The naturopath agreed that Simon was exhibiting behaviors of ADHD and he was sensitive to Simon's feelings in the way that he discussed it, unlike the neurologist. He then advised Katie that children who have ADHD should eliminate corn syrup and food coloring from their diet. These two items are found in many foods and are not easy to eliminate, but it is vital to do so. In addition to corn syrup and food coloring, the naturopath recommended that chocolate and dairy should also be removed from Simon's diet. The dairy was limited to cow's dairy and just the protein. In other words, Simon could still eat goat's cheese and cow's butter, since the butter didn't contain protein just the fat. The naturopath explained that these were sensitivities for Simon, not allergies, but the sensitivities were strong enough to cause him to exhibit ADHD behavior.

In addition to the elimination diet, the naturopath placed Simon on several supplements such as melatonin when Simon has trouble sleeping. Katie gives the melatonin to Simon before bed for only a few days at a time, until his sleep improves. She is careful to stop giving it to him so that his body doesn't become accustomed to it and thus require more and more to be effective. The doctor also gave Simon a calcium and magnesium supplement, an acidophilus supplement to improve his digestion, l-theanine to reduce his anxiety, and GABA to help his sleep and ability to relax. Later, when Simon was about to enter first grade, the naturopath also created an elixir to help calm Simon's anxieties about going back to school, which worked well according to Katie.

It was spring when Katie started Simon on the elimination diet and the supplements. The naturopath doctor advised her that it would take Simon's body about three weeks to clear out the toxins from the offending foods and to begin to use the supplements effectively. Katie and Keith watched and waited. Katie recalls, "It was two and one-half weeks after we started the new diet and the supplements, when Simon's behavior took a turn for the better. We were thrilled. He has now been on this diet for about six months and he is in first grade. His teacher recently told me that she never would have known that he had ADHD if it wasn't in his record."

With relief and newly found belief, Katie happily reports that Simon can now sit long enough to do his worksheets and be patient enough to raise his hand before speaking in class. "Furthermore," she says, "he is socializing much better and has friends both in class and out on the playground. His teacher can motivate him to finish work by rewarding him with more computer time. Plus, although Simon was struggling to read and doing poorly in kindergarten, he is now at the top if his class in reading skills. He is doing *great*."

Katie is thrilled, relieved and thankful for her friends' advice that brought Simon to the naturopath. Despite the improvement, Katie admits, "It isn't easy to follow the elimination diet or give Simon his supplements. Corn syrup and food coloring are in almost all the foods we eat. I never read labels before this experience and it is shocking what is in the foods at the supermarket. It is also hard to get Simon take all of his supplements. I mix them into applesauce to get him to eat them because he can't swallow capsules yet. If I mix too many into the applesauce, it tastes terrible and he won't eat it." Katie loves Simon and notes that he is such a good boy saying, "He always asks me if it is okay to eat something. *He* knows that the new diet makes him happier and improves his ability to concentrate in school." In addition to Simon's own realization that he is now doing better in school, Simon's grandparents on both sides of the family see the improvements in his behavior. It has been a real gift.

CHAPTER 22: RACHELLE'S STORY WITH ASTHMA

Rachelle is a forty-one-year-old mother of two boys, one biological and one adopted from Korea. Prior to having children she was an airplane flight instructor and a pilot. She has stayed at home with her boys during the day and works as a parcel delivery person in the evenings with occasional flying jobs on the weekends. She is intelligent, tall and physically fit, competing in a triathlon just prior to having children. At that time, Rachelle became terribly ill with nausea and her sister suggested that she might be pregnant. During her pregnancy, the nausea persisted strongly. Foods that she ate prior to pregnancy, such as peanut butter, now were repulsive to her. She ate no peanuts whatsoever during her pregnancy or following the birth for at least six months.

Only her first son, her biological son, has food allergies. When he was a baby, he was allergic to dairy, egg, soy, wheat, peanuts, fish, some shellfish and some tree nuts. Rachelle first discovered the symptoms of her son's, Trajan, food allergies when he was just three weeks old. Her family was visiting her new baby and they ordered a pizza. Rachelle was breastfeeding her son. After about one hour, Trajan began to swell and become red all over. Rachelle was perplexed and kept saying to her mother, "He doesn't look right." After a little while, the swelling reduced and he became less red. Later that day, Rachelle brought Trajan to the doctor for a checkup and she explained what had happened. The doctor advised Rachelle not to eat any more dairy while she was breastfeeding. Rachelle complied, although it was a big change for her to eliminate all dairy from her diet. "It was so difficult," she recalls. Rachelle continued to breastfeed Trajan and only introduced solid foods, such as fruits, vegetables and cereals, when he was between eight and nine months old.

Despite her avoidance of dairy, Trajan's skin and health did not improve. He had hives and eczema making his skin red and inflamed. He also had a great deal of mucus in his nose that made breathing difficult for him. Rachelle regularly used the suction to suck out the mucus. In retrospect, Rachelle believes he might have been suffering from either some asthmatic symptoms or some mild anaphylactic symptoms to other foods she was eating. She recalls, "Trajan was sick almost all of the time during his first year of life. I was often up with him at night and got little sleep that year. He was probably sick for twenty-five days of each month." Other contributing factors to his breathing troubles were environmental allergens, including dust. Her husband often swept the floor. Once he swept up the dirt while carrying Trajan in a front pack. Trajan immediately broke out into hives, developed a violent cough and had trouble breathing through the mucus. He developed a respiratory infection by the next morning.

When Trajan was about fifteen months, Rachelle was making meatballs for dinner one evening. Rachelle remembers, "Trajan was clamoring to help. I saw no harm and thought he'd enjoy mixing it up. I sat him on the counter and told him to squish the mixture with his hands. He reached into the bowl of meat, breadcrumbs and egg to mash the mixture. Within seconds he pulled his hands out and screaming. His hands were bright red starting at his wrists all the way to his fingertips. I was shocked and rushed him to the sink and washed his hands furiously over and over. Then slowly the redness began to fade. I didn't call the doctor."

About two months later, when Trajan was seventeen months, Rachelle and her husband took Trajan to Florida to visit family. A cousin was eating a peanut butter and jelly sandwich, and Trajan walked over and touched it. Crying and drooling out the side of his mouth, Trajan ran to his father. Explaining that he did not eat, only touched the sandwich, Rachelle's husband called to her to look at Trajan. Rachelle says, "Trajan just lay in my arms and drooled. My family began to panic and agreed he needed a doctor. We gathered our things quickly and took him out to the car. Once outside, Trajan began breathing deeply and sat up in my arms. I was so relieved that we decided not to go to the doctors after all, but I knew that he was likely allergic to peanuts."

Upon returning home from Florida, Rachelle took Trajan to his regular doctor and explained what had happened. Her pediatric doctor advised her to see an allergist. At the allergist's, Trajan was given a skin prick test on his back. Within a few seconds, each prick swelled up so large that it ran into its neighboring prick and after just minutes Trajan's entire back was swollen and red. Rachelle recalls, "It was terrifying—his entire back blew up and the allergist had to administer the EpiPen® Jr. right there in the office. Then we had to wait for one hour in the office to observe Trajan and make sure nothing more went wrong. The allergist said that he'd seen this happen only one other time in over ten years."

After that scare, the allergist recommended that Trajan undergo an in-office "challenge" test, where he would consume the various foods and the doctor would monitor him for a reaction. Rachelle didn't like this solution for several reasons. First, she already had an idea to which foods he was allergic or at least sensitive. Second, why would she want to endanger her child by directly giving him these foods? Third, this type of testing would take many office visits, at least eight or ten and she began to wonder if the doctor was just "milking" the situation for insurance payments. For these reasons, Rachelle suggested to the doctor that he perform a blood test. But he refused. Rachelle left the office feeling misunderstood and that the doctor wasn't providing a good solution.

A few months later, after Trajan had turned two, it was Thanksgiving and a relative came to visit with their dog. Rachelle requested that the dog remain in the guest's bedroom or outside, rather than roam around the house, in consideration of Trajan's allergies. The guest complied. Upon their departure Rachelle and her husband vacuumed the house to clean out any remaining dog dander. The next day, Trajan started wheezing and became lethargic. He just lay there. Rachelle was distressed and called the pediatric doctor who advised her to come in right away, which she did. At the doctor's office, they found that Trajan was in a full-blown asthma attack. "It blew my mind," reported Rachelle. "I was even more devastated to learn that he had asthma than when I discovered the food allergies." The doctor prescribed a nebulizer breathing treatment, which helped Trajan breath normally.

Rachelle then returned to the allergist for an explanation of the asthma diagnosis. The allergist wanted to put Trajan on more nebulizer treatments. He prescribed five medications for Trajan and gave Rachelle a bag of prescription medications. Rachelle asked how long Trajan would need to use these medications. The allergist replied, "For the rest of his life." Rachelle did not like this solution at all and asked if there were any remedies that were more natural. She remembers, "The mood changed and he interrupted me stating briskly, 'No natural remedies are proven!' then he stormed out of the room. He didn't return, instead sending in the nurse in to finish the appointment by giving me the instructions for all the medications. I was furious. I didn't like his solutions for allergy testing nor asthma treatment. Nor did I like the way he treated me. I vowed never to see that allergist again."

A short time later, when Trajan was two and one-half, Rachelle decided to take him to see a chiropractor who did acupuncture treatments to stimulate Trajan's immune system and kinesiology testing for allergic responses. When the chiropractor tested Trajan for food sensitivities using kinesiology testing, he found that Trajan wasn't showing sensitivity to American cheese, so he wanted to give Trajan a bit. With skepticism she took the tiny piece of cheese on a cracker from the doctor and gave it to Trajan. Rachelle described her son's terrible reaction, "Within seconds, Trajan started crying, his tongue and lips swelled, and he vomited. I brought Trajan outside thinking the fresh air might help as it had in the past. I put him into the car and started to drive to my sister, who was a pharmacist. When I pulled onto the highway, Trajan started projectile vomiting in the back seat. So I pulled over to clean him up. When I took off his dirty shirt and his body was covered with huge silver dollar sized hives."

As fast as she could, she drove to her sister's house and got out of the car screaming, "Help me, help me!" Rachelle took the EpiPen® Jr.

and put it into Trajan's thigh, as her sister read the EpiPen® Jr. instructions. Within seconds the amazing drug worked to stop his reactions and he started to breathe normally. Rachelle called the pediatric doctor's office and explained what had happened. They told her it was good that Trajan vomited because it expelled the cheese from his system, but that she should still go to the emergency room immediately so that Trajan could be monitored. Rachelle was exhausted and both she and Trajan were terribly hungry at the hospital. To make matters worse, she didn't have the allergen-free food that she needed to feed her son and she couldn't trust the hospital's food to be free of dairy and other allergens. A kind nurse helped her by giving them canned fruit. Trajan ate can after can until he had some strength. "It was a nightmarish experience," she painfully remembers.

After that, Rachelle took her son to a dietician who tested Trajan's blood and found it was littered with a variety of unknown substances. The dietician recommended a cleansing diet for Trajan of nothing but chicken, rice and vegetables. After several weeks on this diet, the dietician said that Trajan's blood was much cleaner. Rachelle also found that Trajan, who had been prone to cavities in his teeth, stopped getting them once this strict diet was in place. The dietician advised that previously Trajan had a lot of "bad" bacteria in his gut and probably in his saliva which affected the flora in his mouth causing his teeth to decay. She further explained that there were probably other contributing factors as well. Although his first set of teeth contained many cavities, Trajan's second set of teeth were healthy.

After much trial and tribulations that included three doctors, a dietician, many medications, and a lot of out of pocket cost that the insurance wouldn't cover, Rachelle went to the local health food store for some advice. They recommended a naturopath doctor who might be able to incorporate all the services she wanted. Rachelle gave him a try. At the naturopath's, Trajan, who was now three, was tested for food allergies by both a kinesiology test and a blood test. The naturopath doctor found an interesting anomaly: The test results did not match. The blood test was showing allergens that the kinesiology test did not pick up. The naturopath doctor said he'd never seen this mixed result before. The blood test stated that Trajan was allergic to dairy, eggs, tree nuts, peanuts, fish and shellfish as well as dogs, dust and pollen. The naturopath doctor said Trajan was sensitive to rice, wheat, soy, oat, corn and buckwheat. He recommended that Trajan totally avoid the allergic foods and go on a rotation diet for the sensitive foods. In other words, Trajan could eat rice for one day, then wheat for one day, then soy for one day, and so on. He could also eat meat, fruits and vegetables every day. But he was to avoid dairy, eggs, peanuts, tree nuts, fish and shellfish completely. Rachelle tirelessly adhered to this strict rotation diet for two years.

Her hard work paid off. Although Trajan remains allergic to dairy, eggs, peanuts, black walnuts, some white fish, and shrimp, his food allergies are accurately identified, under control and he is healthy. Furthermore, through a combination of dietary control and exposure to dust, his asthma became manageable. Rachelle reports, "He is no longer on any prescription drugs on a regular basis. The only time he needs any drugs is when he has a serious asthma attack, which usually occurs at the change of each season due to pollen and uncontrollable environmental allergens, weather and humidity."

Rachelle remembers an earlier incident that triggered a terrible asthma episode about a year earlier, "When I was in Florida on vacation, Trajan began to suffer a terrible bout of asthma and weakness after several days of being there. I had to take an emergency flight home, where he recovered. Once home, I learned that the Red Tide came onto the western beaches in Florida from the Gulf making many people sick there. I wonder if the impending Red Tide air caused Trajan to become so ill with his asthma."

Similarly, when Trajan entered preschool, his asthma acted up. Rachelle learned that the rugs in the preschool can carry more cat dander than a home with a cat. Although the school principal was unwilling to replace all of the carpets for financial reasons, a few months later he was forced to when the school was flooded. Again, Trajan's symptoms improved when this environmental allergen was removed.

While the environmental allergens can be difficult to control, there are certain aspects of food that are difficult to control as well, such as chemicals, pesticides and lack of nutrients in our foods. Based upon her own research, Rachelle believes, "The foods we eat are now depleted of nutrients. So many chemicals are used in commercial farms. We should all grow our own food to avoid the chemicals and preservatives in so many of today's foods."

Rachelle has seen the chemicals used on foods. When she was in her early twenties and working as a pilot, she decided to work for a farm in the southern United States. The work involved cornfield dusting with pesticides from the plane. It seemed exciting to her to fly so close to the ground. She and the other pilots watched as the farmer explained how to load the plane with the pesticide.

There was a large metal barrel with the words, "CAUTION" spread all over the side of it. Using gloves, the men picked up the barrel and poured it into the holding tank of the plane. Rachelle watched as the liquid slopped out of the container into the holding tank and mistakenly down the side of the plane, onto the ground, and into the drain in the ground. She again looked at the huge warnings on the side of the barrel and questioned the drippings into the ground to herself. No one wore masks over their faces or eyes. One fellow even picked up the garden hose that had been lying on the ground and drank some water to quench his thirst. When that fellow didn't show up for work over the next three days, the others started to wonder where he might be. On the fourth day, he reappeared. When asked where he was, he said, "I've been in my trailer and couldn't get out of bed. I have been vomiting for three days."

While the poor food quality impacts our children's allergies, family history plays a role as well. Rachelle's father has an almond allergy and Trajan's father was lactose intolerant as a child. Trajan's paternal side of the family also has a history of asthma. With respect to emotional support, Rachelle finds some people are more understanding than others. She recalls, "In the beginning Trajan's grandmother was scared of an allergic reaction so she didn't want to baby sit him while alone. Other people probably think I overreact, but they don't realize that a person can die from food allergies."

Rachelle ponders what good things have come out of these difficult experiences. Now that he is eight, she can reflect on what worked. She says, "I am thankful that I was strong enough emotionally to stand up for Trajan's rights in a non-confrontational way to doctors, teachers and schools. I am also thankful for my husband's full support of me and Trajan in all aspects from emotional support to trying new solutions and to being fully engaged in food avoidance. Also finding the naturopath doctor was great because I think Trajan's improved immune system and growth can be attributed to the supplements and elixirs."

Rachelle feels that Trajan was an amazing child despite the allergies that he has suffered. She explains, "He never went through the terrible twos about which so many other moms complained. He even spoke his first words at only ten months and was an excellent communicator very early."

When Trajan was about five, Rachelle understood his situation well and became confident about how to handle the future. Rachelle thought, "A light bulb went on for me: The world isn't going to revolve around him. He needs to watch out for himself. He needs to know what to do if he has a reaction." She wants Trajan to see that his food allergies are a reality in his life and that he must learn to deal with them assertively and successfully. Now that he is eight, she further considers how to handle his feelings. She feels that it is better for him to sit with other children at a peanut-free table when eating lunch rather than be isolated into a separate room as offered by the school. Rachelle feels like she is over the hump and has passed the worst part of her anger and frustration. She feels positive and proud of how she, her husband and Trajan have handled this difficult situation.

SUMMARY

First and foremost, I hope that reading these interviews helped you feel that you are not alone. By knowing that other people have dealt with food allergy reactions successfully should give you confidence that you can too. Some of the allergic reactions were surprises for the mothers because they had not yet ascertained that their children had food allergies. Other times, the mothers were forced to deal with an accidental dose of the food to which they knew their children were allergic. In all cases, the exposure to the allergen was unintentional.

If there was a non-invasive, safe and reliable way to test children for food allergies, then health care costs, as well as parents' confusion, fear, and frustration would be greatly reduced. Currently, there are blood, skin and muscle tests for allergies. Each has been shown to be unreliable producing either false negative or false positive results. For instance, I recently took my son for blood and skin testing. His blood test results were negative for dairy (*less* than one a scale of one to one hundred) but his skin prick results were positive (three on a scale of one to five). We were so happy for the week between the two tests, when we thought our son had outgrown the allergy. Our allergist said the blood test was a false negative. After the skin test, our allergist told us to avoid dairy for another year.

Other mothers, who have similar experiences, were told by their doctor that the allergy may be gone and to have a "challenge" test in a controlled environment at the doctor's office where the allergy food is fed to the child. My husband and I are left with the decision to either avoid dairy for another year, or to risk a reaction and delayed ability to outgrow the allergy if we "challenge" him by feeding him cow's milk at a different doctor's office.

In summary, after sharing these stories, it is evident that there is a lack of research, evidence and conclusive studies on the causes, testing, and treatments for food allergies. If scientists could accurately predict food allergies in infants, then children could be cared for better. Guessing would be eliminated. Expensive unrelated tests could be avoided. Hospital emergency room visits would be reduced. An ounce of prevention is worth a pound of cure in this situation.

For these reasons, I urge parents and everyone reading this book to write to your congress person, using the sample letter provided in the conclusion, to ask for more funding and research. The Internet address is provided there to save you time in preparing the letter.

In the following section, Theories, Facts and Findings, I provide you with examples of the confusion, some research, possible causes and probable results of food allergies.

Theories, Facts and Findings

CHAPTER 23: MYTHS AND FACTS

Evidence of confusion about food allergies is everywhere. Based upon the interviews in the preceding section and my own research there are different perspectives, beliefs and findings. Here is a sample of the confusion as discussed on the web site of American Family Physician, American Academy of Family Physicians and some others.

Myth #1:   Food allergy is very common.

Fact: Although twenty-five percent of people think they're allergic to certain foods, studies show that about only eight percent of children and two percent of adults has a true food allergy.

Myth #2:   Most people with food allergies are allergic to strawberries and tomatoes.

Fact: Although people can be allergic to any kind of food, most food allergies are caused by tree nuts, peanuts, dairy, eggs, soy, wheat, fish and shellfish.

Myth #3:   Some people are allergic to sugar.

Fact: A condition is called a food allergy when the immune system (the part of the body that fights infections) thinks a certain *protein* in a food is a foreign agent and fights against it. This doesn't happen with sugars and fats.

Myth #4:   Milk allergy is very common in adults.

Fact: Milk allergy is much more common in children than in adults. However, by age six, over eighty percent outgrow the allergy. Symptoms of milk allergy include hives, vomiting and breathing problems after consuming a dairy product. Many adults may experience symptoms similar to milk allergy, as adults often have trouble digesting the sugar in milk. This is called lactose intolerance and is not a true allergy. The symptoms of lactose intolerance are bloating, cramping, nausea, gas and diarrhea.

Myth #5: People with food allergies are allergic to many foods.

Fact: Most people with food allergies are allergic to fewer than four foods.

Myth #6: Food allergy makes people hyperactive.

Fact: The most common sudden symptoms of food allergy are hives (large "bumps" on the skin), swelling, itchy skin, itchiness or tingling in the mouth, a metallic taste in the mouth, coughing, trouble breathing or wheezing, throat tightness, diarrhea and vomiting. There may also be a feeling of impending doom, a feeling that something bad is going to happen, pale skin because of low blood pressure, or loss of consciousness (fainting). The most common chronic illnesses associated with food allergies are eczema and asthma.

Myth #7: Allergy to food dye is common.

Fact: Natural foods cause the most allergic reactions. Studies have found that some food additives, such as tartrazine, or yellow no. 5, and aspartame (brand name: NutraSweet), an artificial sweetener, do cause problems in some people.

Myth #8: Food allergy is either lifelong or is always outgrown.

Fact: Children usually outgrow allergies to milk, eggs, soybean products and wheat. However, people rarely outgrow allergies to peanuts, tree nuts, fish and shellfish.

Myth #9:   Food allergy is not dangerous.

Fact: Food allergy can be fatal if it is severe enough to cause a reaction called anaphylaxis (say: "anna-phil-ax-iss"). This reaction makes it hard for a person to breathe. Fast treatment with a medicine called epinephrine (say: "epp-in-eff-rin") can save your life. If you or your child has a severe allergy, your doctor might give you a prescription for epinephrine self-injection pens. Your doctor can show you how to use them and tell you when to use them. If your doctor thinks you might need to use this medicine, you'll need to carry one with you at all times. A person having an allergic reaction should be taken by ambulance to a hospital emergency room because the symptoms can start again hours after the epinephrine is given. Once a true food allergy is diagnosed, avoid the food that caused it. If you have an allergy, you must read the labels on all the prepared foods you eat. Your allergist can help you learn how to avoid eating the wrong foods. If your child has food allergies, give the school and other caretakers instructions that list what foods to avoid and what to do if the food is accidentally eaten.[16](Myths 1-9)

Myth #10:   Any negative reaction to a food is a food allergy.

Fact: Adverse reactions to food can have many causes. If something does not 'agree with you,' it does not necessarily mean you are allergic to it. Food allergy is a very specific reaction involving the immune system of the body, and it is important to distinguish food allergy from other food sensitivities. Whereas food allergies are rare, food intolerances, which are the other classification of food sensitivities, are more common. Intolerances are reactions to foods or ingredients that do not involve the body's immune system. Intolerance reactions are generally localized, transient and rarely life threatening with one possible exception-sulfite sensitivity. "A good example of a food intolerance is lactose intolerance. And, it is extremely important to know the difference between it and a milk allergy," said Robert K. Bush, M.D., University of Wisconsin. He emphasized that, "Whereas lactose intolerance may result in a bloated feeling or flatulence after consuming milk or dairy products, milk allergy can have life-threatening consequences. The milk allergic patient must avoid all milk proteins."[17]

Myth #11: Breastfeeding can contribute to food allergies.

Fact: There is no solid research showing that women avoiding peanuts during pregnancy or breastfeeding decrease the likelihood of their child to experience allergies. In case of a genetic vulnerability to allergies, exclusive breastfeeding for a minimum of four months can decrease the allergy risk to cow's milk. Breastfeeding for a minimum of three months is effective against wheezing in infants, but there's no solid proof it can impede asthma later. There's no solid proof for the effectiveness of hypoallergenic formulas, when infants are not just breastfed, nor that soy-based formulas can prevent allergies.[18]

Myth #12: There is no cure for food allergies.

Fact: Most medical authorities believe that there is no cure for food allergies because, according to the Food Allergy and Anaphylaxis Network, there are currently no medications that cure food allergies. The fact is, there is certainly much that can be done. A diet that is free of offending foods, together with natural nutritional supplements, enzymes, herbal formulas and homeopathic remedies, can be very beneficial to people with both food allergies and intolerances. Normalizing the digestive function and healing a damaged intestinal lining will go a long way to eliminate adverse food reactions.[19]

CHAPTER 24: TOXIC LOAD THEORY

As I wrote this book I liked to discuss interesting stories from the interviews and research with my husband as we ate our dinner or sat in the whirlpool at our health club on Sunday afternoons. Sometimes I would point out the complexities that people have encountered in the effort to determine to which foods their children are allergic. Many times, my husband would explain his own toxic load theory and how it fits into various situations (he does not have a medical degree). It goes something like this: A child might be allergic to a food or an environmental allergen, but the symptoms wouldn't manifest all of the time, only occasionally or most of the time. Since the symptoms are intermittent, it can be confusing for the parent when trying to ascertain to what foods the child is allergic. The parents of allergic children might point out, "Well, yesterday he had some cheese and was fine, but today he had yogurt followed by a bottle of milk, then vomited." The toxic load theory can explain this because the child may be able to handle a certain amount of these foods without having a reaction. But when given too much, the reaction appears and it can be surprisingly severe.

To further complicate matters, I believe there are other "things" that can cause the toxic load to increase. For instance, the child may be exposed to a genetically modified version of the food this week, as opposed to a more natural version of the same food last week. Or the child might get a dose of pesticides or chemicals by eating a bowl of strawberries that were not washed properly. Further, there might be some environmental allergens in the air, such as pollen in the spring or autumn months which causes the child's immune system to react. We may not even be aware of the load that the child's body is handling, but there may be times when it becomes too much for the child's body and then only a small amount of an additional allergen will send his or her body into a violent reaction.

Also consider the factor of stress on a child's immune system. Most parents send their children to preschool for one to three years prior to starting kindergarten. When children are not in preschool, they are often signed up for gymnastics, ballet, karate, art classes, baseball, or soccer. Parents who keep their children highly active are trying to do the best for their children by training them in skills and keeping their minds busy learning new things. Unfortunately, stress can be created from this constant push to learn, excel and master new skills. Stress can appear when the child has frequent meltdowns because he or she is over tired or over hungry and cannot deal with the next thing. We all know what it feels like to be exhausted and so hungry that your head hurts and you feel weak. This stress can act as another factor in the toxic load on a child's body.

Scientific studies found increased levels of stress in children doing too much. "Daycare or preschool stress can be measured by the levels of cortisol—a stress hormone—that children produce during the day. In normal, healthy people, cortisol levels follow a daily rhythm, peaking when they wake and then falling over the course of the day. Cortisol levels are the lowest just before sleep (Sapolsky 2004). But stress changes the pattern. If you are under stress, your cortisol level rises, regardless of the time of day. In the short term, this helps your body respond to the crisis. But chronic stress, and chronically elevated levels of cortisol, can cause health and developmental problems (Sapolsky 2004). Because cortisol levels are easy to measure in young children, researchers have collected samples from children who attend daycare and children who stay home. In study after study, the results are the same. When children stay home, their cortisol levels show the healthy pattern—rising at waking and decreasing throughout the day. When children attend daycare the pattern changes. Cortisol levels increase during the day (Geoffroy et al 2006). Although it's not entirely clear what aspects of preschool attendance are stressing kids, some possibilities can be ruled out. For instance, it's not about being separated from parents. Kids who receive home-based care do not have elevated cortisol levels, even when their parents are absent (Dettling et al 2000). Nor is it about differences in daytime resting. Kids in group-based childcare show more stress even after taking into account any possible differences in napping or resting opportunities during the day (Watamura et al 2002)."[20]

Similarly, Anthony Kane, M.D. author of, *How to Help the Child You Love,* describes a similar theory of Dr. Doris Rapp, "Food allergies are very difficult to diagnose. One reason is that the symptoms wax and wane. When a child has a classic allergy, for example to bee stings, then every time a bee stings him, he will have a reaction. Food allergies don't work that way. There seems to be a threshold that must be exceeded before there are any symptoms. In addition, this threshold seems to vary from day to day. On some days a food will affect the child, and on other days it won't. Dr. Rapp explains this phenomenon using the analogy of a barrel. We can view each allergic child as if he has a barrel. As long as the barrel is empty or only partially full, your child will have no problems. Your child won't become hyperactive until his barrel is overflowing. Various things will fill your child's barrel. Let's say your child is sensitive to chocolate, cats, and peanut butter. Each of these things all can partially fill his barrel. As long as he only has peanut butter or only plays with the cat, his barrel is only partially full. That means that there are no symptoms and that his behavior is fine. Then one day he has a peanut butter and jelly sandwich, has chocolate ice cream for dessert and plays with the cat all afternoon. These things in combination make his barrel overflow, and by evening he is out of control. Your child has food allergies, but sometimes they affect him and sometimes they don't. The barrel can change sizes. If your child has a cold or is upset, his barrel gets smaller. It takes less to make it overflow. If he is happy his barrel is bigger. It takes more to make it overflow. If he isn't eating well and that day he is low on certain nutrients his barrel gets smaller. Many traditional allergists find this barrel concept ludicrous. It doesn't fit into the pattern of how other allergies work."[21]

For parents who are afraid that they will not expose their children to enough activity if they don't fill their days with social events and classes, consider the following: Day after day of constant activity can actually be detrimental not only to the child's health due to stress but also to their intellectual development. If a child is regularly saying things like, "What are we doing today?" or "Will you play with me?" or "I'm bored," then the child needs to learn the skills of self-entertainment and imaginative play. In other words, keeping our children too active can not only hinder their ability to handle allergies, but may also hinder their ability to learn, create, concentrate, imagine and grow intellectually. By creating an environment at home where a child can explore, question and play, the child *will* learn. One way to discourage this beneficial environment is to constantly scold a child when he or she explores the world outside of his or her set of toys. Allowing the child the freedom to explore in a home environment where dangers have been removed will allow the child to learn and grow naturally.

Some educators support these types of ideas. For instance, The Waldorf Schools believe, "Infants and young children are entirely given over to their physical surroundings; they absorb the world primarily through their senses and respond in the most active mode of knowing: imitation...The environment should offer the child plenty of opportunity for meaningful imitation and for creative play. This supports the child in the central activity of these early years: the development of the physical organism. Drawing the child's energies away from this fundamental task to meet premature intellectual demands robs the child of the health and vitality he or she will need in later life. In the end, it weakens the very powers of judgment and practical intelligence...Through songs and poems [children] learn to enjoy language, to play together, hear stories, see puppet shows, bake bread, make soup, model beeswax, and build houses out of boxes, sheets, and boards. To become fully engaged in such work is the child's best preparation for life. It builds powers of concentration, interest, and a lifelong love of learning." [22]

Therefore, while parents may strive to do the best for their young children by keeping them active, entertained and stimulated, the result may be just the opposite. Children, especially those with allergic tendencies, need less external stimulation, not more. The mind and body will grow naturally if the child is loved and treated kindly.

CHAPTER 25: GENETICALLY MODIFIED FOODS

What is all the fuss about genetically modified foods or "GM" foods? According to Arpad Pusztai, Ph.D., degreed in chemistry and physiology from Budapest and London, respectively, "One of the major health concerns with GM food is its potential to increase allergies and anaphylaxis in humans eating unlabeled GM foodstuffs."[23] These foods have had their DNA changed and can introduce brand new proteins into our bodies.

The following statistics, benefits and drawbacks are from the U.S. Human Genome Project, a thirteen year effort coordinated by the U.S. Department of Energy and the National Institutes of Health. "[I]n 2006, countries that grew ninety-seven percent of the global transgenic crops were the United States (53%), Argentina (17%), Brazil (11%), Canada (6%), India (4%), China (3%), Paraguay (2%) and South Africa (1%)."[24]

Large corporations hire scientists to create these foods so the companies can make more money. Here are the "benefits" to the companies for the genetically modified foods:

Crops: Enhanced taste and quality; reduced maturation time; increased nutrients, yields, and stress tolerance; improved resistance to disease, pests, and herbicides; new products and growing techniques.

Animals: Increased resistance, productivity, hardiness, and feed efficiency; better yields of meat, eggs, and milk; improved animal health and diagnostic methods.

Environment: "Friendly" bioherbicides and bioinsecticides; conservation of soil, water, and energy; bioprocessing for forestry products; better natural waste management; more efficient processing.

Society: Increased food security for growing populations (more food).[25]

But the drawbacks of genetically modified foods include:

Safety: Potential human health impact: allergens, transfer of antibiotic resistance markers, unknown effects.

Potential environmental impact: Unintended transfer of transgenes through cross-pollination; unknown effects on other organisms (e.g., soil microbes); loss of flora and fauna biodiversity.

Access and Intellectual Property: Domination of world food production by a few companies; increasing dependence on industrialized nations by developing countries; biopiracy—foreign exploitation of natural resources.

Ethics: Violation of natural organisms' intrinsic values; tampering with nature by mixing genes among species; objections to consuming animal genes in plants and vice versa; stress for animal.

Labeling: Not mandatory in some countries (e.g., United States); mixing GM crops with non-GM confounds labeling attempts.

Society: New advances may be skewed to interests of rich countries.[26]

Some claim that there are "no genetically modified meat, poultry, dairy or vegetable products on the market."[27] But that doesn't mean animals aren't eating genetically modified foods. Because, in the same breath, "The food industry says if the product has corn or soybeans in it—and most processed foods do—it's probably been genetically modified. Even so, many shoppers have no idea they're already eating the food of the future."[28] Some grassroots groups report that up to seventy percent of food in the grocery store is genetically modified.[29] Now that I know I am probably eating this stuff, and so are my children, what is it and why can it cause reactions?

GMOs are created in a variety of ways. According to Northwest Resistance Against Genetic Engineering, "Beginning in 1996, bacteria, virus and other genes have been artificially inserted into the DNA of soy, corn, cottonseed and canola plants. These unlabeled genetically modified foods carry a risk of triggering life-threatening allergic reactions, and evidence collected over the past decade now suggests that they are contributing to higher allergy rates...In March 1999, researchers at the York Laboratory were alarmed to discover that reactions to soy had skyrocketed by fifty percent over the previous year. Genetically modified soy had recently entered the U.K. from U.S. imports and the soy used in the study was largely GM...The classical understanding of why a GM crop might create new allergies is that the imported genes produce a new protein, which has never before been present. The novel protein may trigger reactions...If the new GM protein is found to contain sequences that are found in the allergen database, according to criteria recommended by the World Health Organization and others, the GM crop should either not be commercialized or additional testing should be done."[30]

I believe we are bombarding our children's bodies with new foods causing their bodies to overreact. Human beings have been around for millions of years. We've thrived on natural foods such as meat, fruits and vegetables. Eating foods that were created in a scientist's lab is sure to have a negative effect on our bodies. It is no wonder that our children's tiny bodies are reacting so violently to these newly invented GM "foods."

According to The Pew Initiative on Food and Biotechnology, "[A] World Health Organization panel released a report on GM foods and allergies, calling for companies to compare amino acid sequences and test protein digestibility. The panel also suggested using blood serum from allergic people to test for potential sensitivity and called for testing new compounds in animal models of allergic reactions. Such models are now under development."[31]

How involved is the United States in this effort? Are we slightly interested or taking a lead role? If finding answers to questions about food allergies helps reduce the cost of healthcare overall, perhaps our federal government could be convinced to increase funding for projects relating to food allergies. Further, if these new foods cause food allergies, let's also ask what other health issues they cause. Could cancer be caused by these test tube foods? Could other problems be on the rise such as autism, ADHD, or asthma because of GM foods?

How can we avoid genetically modified foods? Author Jeffrey Smith writes, "Organic foods are not allowed to contain GM ingredients. Buying products that are certified organic or that say non-GMO [Genetically Modified Organism] are two ways to limit your family's risk from GM foods. Another is to avoid products containing any ingredients from the seven food crops that have been genetically engineered: soy (89%), corn (61%), cottonseed (83%), canola (75%), Hawaiian papaya (50%+) and a little bit of zucchini and crook neck squash. [Numbers in parenthesis are his estimates of genetically modified varieties.] This means avoiding soy lecithin in chocolate, corn syrup in candies, and cottonseed or canola oil in snack foods; dairy products from cows injected with rbGH; food additives, enzymes, flavorings, and processing agents, including the sweetener aspartame (NutraSweet®) and rennet used to make hard cheeses; meat, eggs, and dairy products from animals that have eaten GM feed; honey and bee pollen that may have GM sources of pollen; and contamination or pollination caused by GM seeds or pollen."[32]

When I shop for foods, I find that the organic foods can be a bit more expensive. But if I eliminate most of the expensive pre-packaged foods made with GM ingredients, then it can offset the cost of buying organic, whole foods, such as fruits and vegetables. Parents often complain that their children won't eat anything but macaroni and cheese or their favorite crackers. But if you eliminate these foods from your home (donate them or toss them) and stop buying them, an act that takes determination and courage, your children will eventually eat the foods that you want them to eat. Children will surely complain for a week or two, but eventually they will get hungry enough to eat the foods that are available to them. Reassuring yourself that you are doing the best for your children will help you get over the period of change. Eventually their tastes for foods will change and they will crave the healthier foods. This is a gift that you can give your children for the rest of their lives. When they are adults, they will choose an apple for a snack instead of a fruit pie sitting in a vending machine for weeks, or longer.

CHAPTER 26: PESTICIDES, ANTIBIOTICS, HORMONES

Pesticides

According to a report entitled, "Pesticide Residue Regulation: Analysis of Food Quality Protection Act Implementation," in 1996 when the Food Quality Protection Act was enacted, there were 9,728 residue tolerance levels and exemptions for pesticide ingredients. Of these there were 1,691 organophosphate pesticide ingredients that were sprayed on fruit trees, vegetables, ornamental plants, cotton, corn, soybeans, rice, and wheat to kill boll weevils or fruit flies. But by 2002, once the EPA assessed them, they revoked 703 of them because they were found to have a highly variable, toxic effect on the nervous systems of people and other animals...some are acutely toxic...risking damage to developing brains and nervous systems.[33]

Our nervous system is apparently linked to our digestive system and thus food allergies. According to the Allergy Society of South Africa, "Systems which may be involved in food allergy are the skin, respiratory (breathing) organs and the central nervous system."[34] Similarly, J.D. Woods and others at Ohio State University discovered, "that signaling between mast cells and the ENS [enteric nervous system] underlies intestinal...anaphylactic responses associated with food allergies."[35] In other words, she is demonstrating how the digestive and nervous systems are linked. Woods later recommends in 2006 that, "[N]eurogastroenterological research must determine whether presynaptic inhibition in the ENS has the same significance for the common symptoms of food allergy, mucosal inflammation, and brain-gut interactions in stress in humans, as is known to exist in animal models."[36] In summary, researchers have found evidence that pesticides can damage our central nervous system and the nervous system contributes to how we react to foods. So we need to ask, if animals have allergic reactions to pesticides in foods, do humans react similarly? Consequently, if we find something to help the animals, can it help humans too?

Since the organophosphate pesticides were in our homes, hands and mouths for at least six years from 1996 to 2002, we need to ask, of the remaining allowed pesticides, when will researchers learn whether the harm that they cause to our bodies also causes us to be allergic to foods? It is up to us, the consumers, to ask our government's agencies this question because so many companies' pocketbooks are affected by pesticide production. According to EPA, there are approximately thirty major pesticide producers, 100 smaller producers, 2,500 formulators, 29,000 distributors and retailers, 40,000 commercial pest control firms, 1 million farms, and 3.5 million farm workers. All of these companies and people would be affected by pesticide regulations.[37] We can't expect all of these companies and people to self-regulate because it would cost them money and would reduce their profits when dangerous pesticides are outlawed. It is up to us to ask our government to improve regulations and safety for our sake and that of our children.

Antibiotics and Hormones

Farmers use antibiotics and hormones to increase the growth and milk output of cows. But there are probably unintended negative consequences associated with these additives. Specifically, could the antibiotics and hormones fed to livestock affect our bodies' allergic responses to the foods we eat?

One study shows that when given a more natural form of cow's milk, allergies in children were less. "A large European study of nearly 15,000 children revealed that drinking farm milk (unpasteurized milk produced from grazing cows) rather than commercial milk (pasteurized milk from large factory-farm-fed cows) is linked with a lower risk of asthma and allergies. Children who drank farm milk at any time of their lives had a twenty-six percent lower risk of asthma, thirty-three percent lower risk of pollen sensitivity, and a remarkable *fifty-seven percent* lower risk of food allergies. This was true for children who lived on a farm and those who lived in the city and drank farm milk. It was not clear from the study whether the reduction in risk was due to the fact that the milk was unpasteurized or the fact that the farm milk came from grazing cows. Milk from cows raised on pasture has more omega-3 fatty acids, antioxidants, and other nutrients that may reduce the risk of allergies."[38] Could our children's bodies be affected by the antibiotics loaded into commercial beef and milk thereby causing either allergies to antibiotics or foods like dairy?

Unlike organic farm milk, most of our grocery store milk is from cows which are given antibiotics. "Factory-Farm proponents suffered a major blow…as the Union of Concerned Scientists released an important study in Washington D.C. by Charles Benbrook and Margaret Mellon showing that seventy percent of all antibiotic drugs in the U.S. are being fed to farm animals as growth promoters or production aids. The study, which generated significant headlines and TV coverage across the nation, points out that twenty-five million pounds of valuable antibiotics— roughly seventy percent of total U.S. antibiotic production—are fed to chickens, pigs, and cows every year for non-therapeutic purposes like growth promotion. The drug-dependent U.S. meat industry has tried to downplay its massive use of antibiotics—a practice which is now starting to be banned in Europe—claiming that it was using *only* eighteen million pounds a year of antibiotics in animal feed each year."[39] Perhaps the United States is trailing Europe in understanding the negative results of using so many antibiotics and hormones. We need to ask our government to set some limits on the use of antibiotics. We need to ask, "What are the ramifications of these antibiotics on our children?"

Another way that farmers increase the milk production is by using Bovine Growth Hormone (BGH). Once cows are given BGH so much milk is produced that it often causes the cows' udders to get infected. Once the udders are infected, the cows are given even more antibiotics. Then when the cow is milked, a pus-like substance is found in their milk. This pus is made up of bacterial infection and antibiotic drugs. Then people drink it. "U.S. farmers use Bovine Growth Hormone to boost milk output. Some [of these] cows have produced more than *thirty tons* of milk in a year. Up to half of American dairy cows suffer BGH-induced mastitis, an excruciating inflammation and bacterial infection of the udder...[and] are treated with antibiotics...Antibiotics are passed to humans who drink cow's milk. One-third of milk products are contaminated with antibiotic traces."[40]

Some countries outside of the United States have decided to no longer allow the use of Bovine Growth Hormone. "BGH is banned in both Canada and Europe. BGH-treated cows are also more likely to contract mastitis, a persistent infection of the cows' udders. These cows are then treated with a myriad of antibiotics and sulfa drugs. Trace amounts of these drugs as well as pus and bacteria from the infected udders are also found in their milk."[41]

There is evidence that these trace antibiotics can effect allergic reactions in people. "Many of these antibiotics, even in trace amounts, can cause allergic reactions—from mild reactions such as hives to anaphylactic shock."[42] Perhaps it isn't primarily the dairy proteins to which so many children appear to be allergic, but instead the antibiotics and infection pus in the milk.

CHAPTER 27: DELAYED ALLERGIC REACTIONS

The majority of examples and stories in this book are about children who can go into anaphylactic shock if they consume the food to which they are allergic. But there are other ways that a food allergy can manifest that might affect behavior. In fact, some scientists believe that autism, attention-deficit-hyperactivity-disorder (ADHD) and asthma could be related to food allergies.

An article entitled, "Food Allergy Testing for ADHD and Autism," reports that, "[A] groundbreaking paper on this topic entitled Allergy and Learning Disabilities in Children in Annals of Allergy in March 1976...took note of the 'allergic tension-fatigue syndrome observed by Speer' and noted that it was a 'symptom complex accepted by many allergists.' They then went on, using both scratch test and intradermal techniques (which means 'injecting allergy-provoking substances beneath the skin to see if there is an allergic reaction') and were able to positively correlate food allergies associated with IgE allergic reactions with actual changes in IQ scores. In other words, the more the food allergies, the lower the IQ scores in the children tested. The lower the food allergies, the higher the IQ scores in the children tested. This was truly a groundbreaking piece of work."[43]

This test shows that the foods we eat affect the way we feel and think. If our children are eating foods that they cannot digest properly because they are allergic to these foods, then it can affect their mind. Just like when we drink coffee, we might feel quicker mentally, as opposed to when we drink alcohol, we might feel slower mentally. Our brains can be affected by the foods we eat.

Sometimes the effect is quick, other times it occurs the next day. There are two types of antibodies created: IgE and IgG. The IgE appears right away and is visible with a skin prick test. But the IgG antibody might not appear for a day or two after eating the offending food. (I use the following to remember the difference: IgE means immediate; IgG means gradual.) Since the IgG is a gradual response, it makes it harder to test for the IgG antibody. Furthermore, it makes it harder to see the link between the offending food and its effect. It seems possible that foods which cause some children to have an IgG antibody might affect the child's brain so he or she might exhibit autism or ADHD, or the lungs causing asthma.

An article entitled, "Food Allergy and Lung Disease," reports that, "Delayed patterns of food allergy can cause chronic asthma and/or bronchitis and are among the most neglected causes of chronic or 'intrinsic' asthma. Diet revision can resolve chronic asthma...Patients with delayed pattern food allergy have the most persistent inflammatory form of chronic asthma. Skin tests do not show delayed patterns of food allergy and diet revision must be complete and comprehensive to resolve this common form or allergic asthma...Food allergens may be found in the blood stream in circulating immune complexes that trigger the release of immune mediators in the bloodstream. These chemicals cause a variety of symptoms, including constriction of the bronchial smooth muscle in the lungs; this is the first event of an asthmatic attack."[44] In other words, I interpret this to mean that just like a child's tongue or lips may swell, his or her lung muscle may be affected by the foods they eat. Just because we cannot see the lungs, it doesn't mean they aren't swelling or changing because of an allergic reaction.

In the next three chapters, I explore the evidence and possibilities that these delayed food allergy reactions may cause or contribute to the disorders of autism, ADHD and asthma.

CHAPTER 28: FOOD ALLERGIES AND AUTISM

The rate of autism in children (aged six to twenty-one) has increased from 5,415 (1991/1992) to 118,602 (2001/2002) to 300,000 (2006).[45][46] Furthermore, *late* onset autism (starting in the second year) was almost unheard of in the 1950s, 1960s, and 1970s—but today such cases outnumber *early* onset cases five to one. [47]

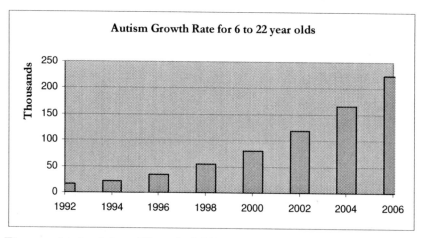

Figures obtained from Thoughtful House Center for Children.[48]

The remainder of this chapter is a description of how an autistic child might be affected by food allergies. This material is taken from an article that I wrote for San Diego Family Magazine. It is reprinted here with permission.[49] (Slight modifications have been made to bring the information up-to-date.)

Parents want the best for their children. If there was a chance to improve the behavior of an autistic child, these parents are eager to try. Even though a cure for autism doesn't exist, what if there was a drug-free way to improve a child's chance for a better life? Specifically, is there something that can be done to reduce autistic behavior in a child? There may be. There is evidence that some (or many) autistic children are allergic to foods and that those allergic reactions do not result in the normal response of anaphylactic shock, hives, or vomiting but instead produce autistic behavior. Indeed, some parents have successfully reduced or eliminated the autistic behavior of their child by eliminating certain foods.

Step outside the world of autism for a moment and into the world of an addict. New reality TV shows now let us see "interventions" of people who are addicted to drugs or alcohol. It is clear to friends and family that the behavior of their loved one is being affected by the drugs or alcohol. Detoxification of the body from drugs or alcohol is demanded by the family and friends for their loved one to return to a normal and healthy behavior.

Step back into the world of autism. What if there was a drug-like substance that affects the autistic child's brain to cause autistic behavior? If that drug-like substance were removed, would the child's brain recover, at least partially, from the autistic behavior? In other words, is something that the child is ingesting which causes his or her brain to react thereby triggering the autistic behaviors?

In lay person's terms, sometimes food can enter the bloodstream before being fully digested. The food can enter the bloodstream through holes in the intestine caused by an overgrowth of candida or because it cannot be fully digested due to the lack of sufficient enzymes. The body sees the undigested food in the bloodstream as a foreign invader and sends the immune system to the rescue. For children with autism, this allergic response of the body "set[s] off a chain of events resulting in the production of psychoactive chemicals that affect brain function, possibly by creating opioid-like hallucinogenic substances that act on the brain in a toxic manner," according to researcher Alan Friedman.[50]

Therefore, by removing the offending food (allergen), the body may stop sending the chemicals that affect the brain, which can in turn stop its response of producing autistic behavior. Mother and author, Karyn Seroussi, reports that after changing her son's diet, "What happened next was nothing short of miraculous. Miles stopped screaming, he didn't spend as much time repeating actions, and by the end of the first week, he pulled on my hand when he wanted to go downstairs. For the first time in months, he let his sister hold his hands to sing 'Ring Around a Rosy'....[A]s each day passed, Miles continued to get better. A week later, when I pulled him up to sit on my lap, we made eye contact and he smiled."[51]

So which foods might cause autistic behavior? The most popular food offenders for autism appear to be dairy, wheat, gluten, caffeine, chocolate, artificial colors or flavors, soy, and corn, but there may be others. Elimination of one or two food allergens at a time, with a watchful eye to see results, is the best approach. "Many parents report a casein-free (dairy protein) and gluten-free diet increases eye contact, attention, and mood while decreasing aggressive or oppositional behavior, tantrums, and poor attention. Theories for improvement of casein-free diet include improved brain function due to removal of cow's milk protein by-products that have opiate like effects. Casomorphin is protein fragment or peptide sequence derived from casein that is considered to have an opiate like effect. There are several casomorphins produced by digestion of casein from cow's milk. People who stop eating wheat and dairy containing foods commonly report withdrawal symptoms."[52]

Eliminating even one of these food allergens is not any easy task, but the effort could be well worth it. For instance, dairy is prevalent in most packaged foods including bread, crackers, cookies and cakes. Dairy can be tricky to eliminate because it can be disguised under names such as casein, whey, lactic acid, potassium caseinate, lactalbumin, lactate, galactose and a few other names. Parents need to research each allergen that they want to eliminate to learn under what names that allergen might appear and in which foods. The chapter entitled "Identify the Big Eight Allergens" can help with this task. Research can effectively be done on the Internet and by checking with an allergist.

Another challenge can be proving that the allergy exists. The normal skin prick testing which locates an IgE antibody may not work for this type of situation—there will be no swelling of the skin prick test site. Instead, the allergist might need to look for the delayed reaction IgG antibody in the blood, which may take a day or two to form after ingesting the food.

There is some good news on identifying allergens on food labels. New laws have been put into place by the USDA, specifically the Food Allergen Labeling and Consumer Protection Act of 2004 (FALCPA) which became effective January 1, 2006, "Under FALCPA, food labels are required to state clearly whether the food contains a 'major food allergen.' The law identifies as a major food allergen any of eight allergenic foods: Dairy; eggs; fish such as bass, flounder, and cod; crustacean shellfish such as crab, lobster, and shrimp; tree nuts such as almonds, walnuts, and pecans; peanuts; wheat; and soybeans. The law also identifies as a major food allergen any ingredient that contains protein derived from any of these eight foods. The plain language declaration requirement of FALCPA also applies to flavorings, colorings, and incidental additives that are or contain a major food allergen."[53]

But some challenges exist in that other allergens, which may affect autistic children, are not required to be displayed as clearly as these top eight allergens, listed above. For instance, gluten, caffeine, and corn would not be set forth in any special manner but rather may just appear as ordinary ingredients in the list. Additionally, products that were packaged prior to January 1, 2006, that may still be "on the shelf" will not carry the allergen label. Further, products that are packaged out of the country may not adhere to these labeling laws.

Although there are no conclusive studies to prove that autistic behavior can be reduced by eliminating allergens, there is plenty of testimonial evidence. Why not give a child a chance at a better life by eliminating possible allergens from his diet and watching the results?

CHAPTER 29: FOOD ALLERGIES AND ADHD

In 2006, the Centers for Disease Control and Prevention's (CDC) National Health Interview Survey stated, "Four and one-half million children three to seventeen years of age (seven percent) had Attention Deficit Hyperactivity Disorder (ADHD). Boys were more than twice as likely as girls to have ADHD (ten and four percent respectively)." [54]

They also found that white children with lower incomes and poor health were more likely to suffer from ADHD. Symptoms include inattention, hyperactivity, impulsivity, academic underachievement, or behavior problems, all or part of which have been harmful for the child academically or socially for at least six months. The diagnoses are always made based upon behavior, since no laboratory or imaging tests can determine if a child has ADHD.

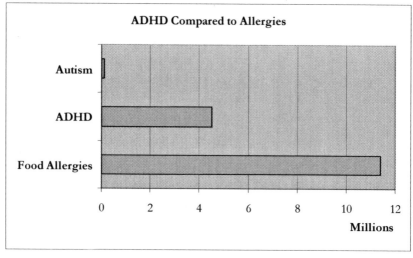

Based upon figures in 2006.

In 2005, it was reported by the CDC that of the four and one-half million diagnosed about one-half are taking medication for ADHD. [55] I think we all agree that medications can have negative side effects. According to Anthony Kane, MD author of, *How to Help the Child You Love,* "Treating the food sensitivities in ADHD children has a number of advantages over using medication. One major advantage [is that all of] the current methods of treatment can be used to treat preschool children. Most clinicians do not use medication on preschool children. A more significant advantage of treating food allergy is that when it works, it works all day. In contrast, Ritalin wears off in about four hours."[56] Furthermore, "a study by the federal government's National Toxicology Program (NTP) found that doses of Ritalin that only modestly exceeded the maximum recommended dose in humans caused liver tumors in mice. 'Millions of young children take Ritalin for years on end, and children may be especially susceptible to a carcinogen's effects,' says Samuel Epstein, a cancer expert at the School of Public Health at the University of Illinois."[57]

Some research has been done on what foods tend to affect ADHD children. "[In the early] 1970s, Dr. Benjamin Feingold, then chief emeritus of the Department of Allergy at the Kaiser Foundation Hospital and Permanente Medical Group in San Francisco, reported a link between diet and several physical and allergic conditions. Thirty to fifty percent of Feingold's hyperactive patients said they benefited from diets free of artificial colorings and flavorings, and certain natural chemicals (salicylates found in apricots, berries, tomatoes, and other foods)."[58]

According to the Center for Science in the Public Interest, "[W]hen children [are] on a modified diet from which dyes were excluded....the behavior of up to eighty-eight percent of the children improved significantly...When the children consumed cookies with the dyes, some children showed markedly worse behavior...[Furthermore, the exclusion diet is a] diet that exclude[s] dyes, milk, chocolate, citrus fruit, and other foods suspected of affecting behavior. Sixty-two subjects (eighty-two percent) responded favorably to dietary modification [which]...led the researchers to conclude that all of those sixty-two children were affected adversely by tartrazine, benzoic acid (a food preservative), milk, wheat, oranges, eggs, and chocolate."[59] The modified diet needs to run for two to three weeks for the body to clear out the allergens previously in the body, before results are visible.

Because there are many foods to which a child with ADHD can be allergic, determining which foods to eliminate can be a challenge. For instance, if he is allergic to five foods, then by successfully eliminating one of these five, his behavior may improve only a little. If all five foods are successfully eliminated, then his behavior might improve significantly. You can try to eliminate one food at a time, and in that way determine what the improvement is for each and every food. But it can become frustrating because the process can take a long time of experimenting, which can be tiring for both the parent and the child.

Furthermore, addictive cravings and withdrawal symptoms are said to exist in many food allergy patients when they stop eating the offending foods. "It has been suggested that this may be because some protein fragments formed when food is broken down are similar to endorphins, which the body produces naturally to counteract pain and produce euphoria. Then the allergy sufferer's body becomes adapted to that level of endorphin activity and so craves the allergen in order to maintain the endorphin levels."[60]

Another method to ascertain food allergies for a child with ADHD is to visit a pediatric allergist who can test for food allergies. But the regular skin prick tests that locate the IgE antibody, may not work for children with ADHD because their reaction is delayed. In regular skin prick tests an IgE antibody is created almost immediately upon coming into contact with the allergen, making the skin rise up in bump. But children with ADHD might not have this kind of allergic response. "IgG-mediated food allergies are delayed immune reactions to foods which can occur anywhere from a few hours to a few days after exposure to the reactive foods."[61] It makes sense that the allergic response by the body is delayed, since the behavior of ADHD doesn't always occur immediately (within minutes) after consuming the offending food. Unfortunately, this delayed reaction adds to the complexity of identifying to what foods the

ADHD child is reacting. In these cases an IgG antibody is created so the allergist must test for the delayed reaction IgG antibody in the blood. Sometimes the RAST blood tests are not reliable either and some doctors recommend having the testing done twice to improve the accuracy of the results. Even conducting the test by two different labs and at two different times may increase the accuracy of the results.[62]

Despite the difficulty of identifying allergens, eliminating foods to improve ADHD behavior could be well worth the effort for both the parent and the child. "Some parents who've put their children on special diets, though, say their children willingly cooperate in making dietary changes, especially after they discover that those changes make them feel better. Some older children avidly read labels to avoid certain ingredients."[63]

CHAPTER 30: FOOD ALLERGIES AND ASTHMA

According to the American Academy of Allergy Asthma and Immunology, "Between 1980 and 1994, the number of children who have asthma has increased 160% while adults increased 75%. Twenty million Americans have asthma in 2005 and almost one-half, about nine million, children had asthma in 2002. Every day roughly eleven people die due to asthma and a reported 5,000 deaths occur each year. The incidence of asthma is about one-third higher in African Americans than whites and one-third higher in females than males."[64]

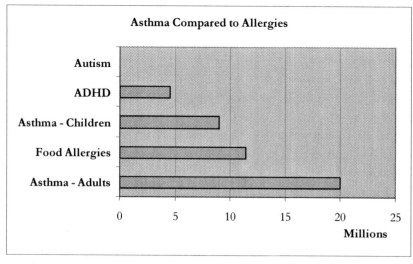

Based upon figures from 2002 to 2006.

Asthma patients often treat the symptoms of their attacks with medication. These medications can have long-term and short-term negative side effects such as fogginess and fatigue. But preventing the attack through eliminating food allergies could be the answer to all the side-effects of medication.

One of the symptoms of a true food allergy is eczema. Eczema, also referred to as atopic dermatitis, is often suffered by those with asthma.

"Asthma symptoms such as coughing, wheezing, or difficulty breathing due to narrowed airways, may be triggered by food allergy, especially in infants and children."[65]

Dr. Greene believes, "Most children with life threatening asthma also have food allergies, according to a fascinating study published in the July 2003 Journal of Allergy and Clinical Immunology—the first study to show that food allergies are a risk factor for severe asthma in children. Perhaps food allergies make asthma worse, or perhaps asthma makes food allergies worse. I expect that both are true. About four to eight percent of children with known asthma are known to have food allergies. Among those with asthma severe enough to place them in an ICU on ventilators, 52.6 percent have food allergies, especially to peanuts or nuts. Food allergies in children are often overlooked."[66]

If food allergies are linked to asthma then why isn't it more obvious when an asthma attack follows ingesting the offending food? Dr. D.G. Wraith, consultant physician with the Allergy Clinic in London states, "Food allergy is a very important cause of asthma but is often over-looked. It is important because it may cause severe symptoms and asthma still has a high mortality despite improvements in drug therapy. It is overlooked because the usual skin tests are often negative and the history is often not helpful as symptoms appear gradually hours or days after ingestion of the food. IgE and Non-IgE mechanisms can cause asthma. Patients with no positive skin tests were shown to react to foods. In Wraith's studies, milk, wheat, egg, yeast, preservatives, color-ings, coffee and cheese were the main foods implicated. Other manifes-tations of food allergy are typical in sixty-five percent of the asthmatic patients."[67]

It may be difficult to link the food allergies to the asthma attack, because as with ADHD and autism, the reaction may not be immediate. When reactions occur several hours or two days later it is not the typical IgE antibody, but rather the IgG antibody. As described earlier in the chapters on autism and ADHD, identifying food allergies for a child with asthma may not work with the traditional skin prick tests because the IgE antibody must affect the skin within about twenty minutes. Instead, the IgG antibody may not appear for a day or two, so a lab analysis of the blood to identify an IgG antibody would be needed. Sometimes the blood tests are not reliable and some doctors recommend having the testing done twice to improve the accuracy of the results. Again, even conducting the test by two different labs and at two different times may increase the accuracy of the results.[68]

Despite the difficulty in identifying and eliminating foods to improve asthma, it might just be the best answer. Here is an interesting example from NPTech Services in the United Kingdom:

> Christian Mayer, world class athlete, is among the benefactors of the attention given to the relationship between food intolerance and respiratory problems. This Austrian skier, who won the World Cup in the Giant Slalom two years in a row and a bronze medal at the Winter Olympics in Lillehammer, suffered every season with breathing problems.
>
> The stuffy air in airplanes and hotels exacerbated his condition when he had to travel to competitions. Needless to say, his coach was not happy about having one of his top skiers waylaid by a health problem. He sent Christian to an Austrian physician, Dr. Stephen Shimpf, who specializes in immunotherapy and preventative medicine in Salzburg. As he does with many of his patients, Dr. Shimpf tested Christian for food intolerance.
>
> The results of the blood test showed that the skier was intolerant to rice, milk products, wheat, apples, bananas, and beer most of which he consumed every day. Once he removed those foods his stuffy nose cleared up. In addition, he was able to avoid (unlike some of his team members) the usual seasonal colds and flu. As an added bonus he lost the extra ten pounds he typically gained in the off-season and he had more energy.

But this world-class athlete says the most important benefit is this, "I'm winning. Right after the test I won my first World Cup in America. I was surprised by the test results because I'd always thought foods like apples and bananas are healthy, but they're not for me. I avoid my reactive foods and I feel better."

Dr. Shimpf, however, was not surprised by the results, "I've got used to great results with food intolerance testing with my patients, so amazing results like this no longer astonish me."[69]

CHAPTER 31: FOOD ALLERGIES AROUND THE WORLD

Introduction

It appears the most impressive research cooperation that has been organized is the EuroPrevall study of food allergies which accepted the following participating countries: Italy, Switzerland, Iceland, Ghana, Germany, Lithuania, Spain, Austria, Sweden, Bulgaria, the Netherlands, United Kingdom, Denmark, Poland, Greece, France, New Zealand, Australia, Russia, India and China.

"In June 2005, the work of the European Union (EU) Integrated Project EuroPrevall was started. EuroPrevall is the largest research project on food allergy ever performed in Europe. Major aims of the project are to generate for the first time reliable data on the prevalence of food allergies across Europe and on the natural course of food allergy development in infants. Improvement of in vitro diagnosis of food allergies is another important aim of the project. The present review summarizes current knowledge about the clinical presentation of food allergy and critically reviews available diagnostic tools at the beginning of the project period. A major problem in diagnosis is a relatively poor 'clinical specificity' i.e. both positive skin tests and in vitro tests for specific IgE are frequent in sensitized subjects without food allergy symptoms. So far, no in vitro test reliably predicts clinical food allergy. EuroPrevall aims at improving the predictive value of such tests by proceeding from diagnosis based on allergen extracts to purified allergen molecules, taking into account the affinity of the IgE-allergen interaction, and evaluating the potential of biological in vitro tests such as histamine release tests or basophil activation tests including assays performed with permanently growing cell lines."[70]

I contacted EuroPrevall to inquire as to whether the United States declined to join and learned, "EuroPrevall is only in Europe, with some expansion to developing countries in Asia and Africa. It was not the in-tent of this project to expand to the U.S.," according to Doreen McBride, MBA, Academic Researcher, Project Coordinator, Institute for Social Medicine, Epidemiology and Health Economics, Charité University Medical Center, 10098 Berlin, Germany.

We need to ask our federal government to become more fully engaged in researching food allergies in the U.S. like in Europe. The rates are increasing and will likely continue to increase. Currently one in thirteen children has food allergies in the U.S.—about six to eight percent of children and four percent of adults. We are not alone—food allergies exist around the world. Here are some facts.

Australia

"The prevalence of anaphylaxis in Australia is estimated to be one in 100 people." Common food allergies: "Milk, peanuts, shellfish, eggs, tree nuts, fish, sesame, and soy. Under the new FSANZ Food Standards Code as of 2002, wheat, gluten-containing cereals, crustacea, eggs, fish, milk, tree nuts, sesame seeds, peanuts, soy, and sulfites must be named on the ingredient list at all times without exception)," per the Food Allergy and Anaphylaxis Network and Anaphylaxis Australia.[71]

Canada

"One to two percent of the general population are considered to be at risk for anaphylaxis, and the number is higher among children (two to eight percent)." Common food allergies: "Peanuts, tree nuts (almonds, hazelnuts, cashews, walnuts, etc.), soy, sesame seeds, wheat, milk, eggs, fish, shellfish, and sulfites. The priority allergens must be listed on the label or the product is subject to recall. The primary ingredients are listed by name except for oils (with the exception of peanut oil), fats, colors, and flavors. It is proposed and recommended that the plant source be identified by common name for each of the following foods: hydrolyzed plant protein, flour, gluten, starch and modified starch. This is not, however, a regulation. Labeling exemptions under the Food and Drug Regulations still include: Seasonings, flavorings, colors, some

items less than five percent or ten percent, cross contact during processing, source of domestic oils (except peanut, which must be declared), hydrolyzed plant protein, lecithin and starch)," per the Food Allergy and
Anaphylaxis Network and Anaphylaxis Canada and Association Quebe-
coise des Allergies Alimentaires.[72]

China

According to Children's Hospital Affiliated to Chongqing Medical
University , a study of 119 infants with food allergies showed that, the
cumulative tolerance probabilities of cow's milk and egg were forty-two
and thirty-one percent one year after diagnosis respectively, sixty-three
and sixty-two percent two years later, seventy-seven and eighty percent
three years later, and one hundred percent after four years. Their conclusion stated that at least seventy-five percent of children with egg or
cow's milk allergy could develop tolerance to egg or cow's milk within
three years after diagnoses. It also showed an increase incidence of
other ailments. Specifically, of these children almost eleven percent also
suffered from another food allergy; about twelve percent also suffered
from asthma; about three percent also suffered from allergic rhinitis.[73]
"In...China, rice allergy is more common."[74] "In the United States and
China, per-capita consumption of peanuts is the same, but China has
virtually no peanut allergies. One difference: We eat mostly dry-roasted
peanuts, even in peanut butter; the Chinese eat peanuts either boiled or
fried. The higher temperatures from dry roasting appear to expose more
allergens in the peanuts, Sampson says."[75]

China's Dr. Xiu-Min Li is collaborating with Hugh Sampson, MD at
Mt. Sinai on a Chinese herbal remedy project that has shown peanut
allergic mice given this mixture for one month were completely protected from peanut induced anaphylaxis for six months. There are two
mixtures being tested: "Food Allergy Herbal Formula-2 (FAHF-2)" and
"Butanol-Purified FAHF-2."

As of September 2006 the studies have found that:

- the first mixture, FAHF-2, tastes bitter so is difficult to administer it to children, but it was shown to have "excellent efficacy and safety profiles."

- the second mixture, Butanol-Purified FAHF-2, is difficult to manufacture for "human use in an industrial setting."

Continued research, testing, clinical trials and manufacturing for both products for use in adults are ongoing and planned as required by the FDA.[76]

France

"A survey was [given] to estimate the prevalence of food allergies. The second goal was to determine the main characteristics of the allergies. About seven percent had true food allergies. The main foods reported as causing adverse reactions were cow's milk, eggs, kiwis, peanuts, fish, tree nuts, and shrimp. Cow's milk, eggs, and peanuts were the main foods reported as causing allergies. Exotic fruits, shellfish, and tree nuts appeared to be relatively new allergens," per Allergologie-Pneumologie, Hôpital des Enfants, Toulouse Cedex, France.[77]

Germany

"As of 2006, the main allergy-causing foods during childhood are cow's milk and hen's eggs, fish, soy, wheat, peanuts, and nuts. Coupled with a familial predisposition (atopy), a food allergy can lead to neurodermatitis, hay fever and bronchial asthma. Peanuts, fish, hen's eggs and cow's milk are important food allergens for adults, too. However, allergic reactions to hen's egg and cow's milk often disappear in the first years of life. Sufferers of pollen allergy have developed allergic reactions to celery, spices, nuts and some types of fruit more frequently in recent years. The observed rise in food allergies can thus be explained by the parallel increase in the number of people who are allergic to pollen. Food allergy sufferers react to certain foods throughout their lives. The food allergy is triggered by contact with the allergy-causing food and the formation of IgE-type antibodies, the immunological reaction. Renewed contact triggers the allergic symptoms. Foods that can cause a pollen-associated allergic reaction have a related structure and a similar protein design (high sequence identity) to the allergic ingredients in pollen. That's why these foods trigger a food allergy in individuals who are allergic to pollen. In Central Europe two to three percent of adults and four percent of infants have food allergies. The proportion of the infant group with dermatitis is even as high as thirty percent," per BfR Federal Institute for Risk Assessment.[78]

India

"Allergy can develop to almost any food, but some foods are more allergenic. Allergies vary from region to region depending upon the availability of the food item processing and eating habits. Allergy to sea food (shrimp, lobster, prawn, crab, mollusks) is seen in coastal areas and in land-locked areas where seafood is freely available. Similarly, allergy to fish is seen in areas where it is eaten frequently. Animal milk (cow, buffalo), egg and wheat are common food allergens. Dals or lentils (such as mash lentils, arhar or yellow lentils, channa or Bengal lentils and rajmah or French beans) have been reported to cause allergy in some patients in India. Peanuts and tree nuts (almond, walnut, etc) are also allergenic to some. Fruits and some food additives may produce symptoms. Allergy can develop to foods which were tolerated earlier. Reactions to nuts and seafood tend to be more severe. Fortunately, milk and egg allergies disappear with age in most children, but other allergies persist."[79]

"Although there has been a great concern in western countries about food allergies, in India the prevalence of food allergy although preserved has not been systematically studied. Unfortunately, there is not much awareness about food hypersensitivity reaction in India. Indian food is quite complex and it is necessary for a high risk person to know to what kind of food he is allergic. Diagnosis of food allergy is a quite lengthy procedure and many times it is not possible to avoid the offending food. There has been a great concern in many countries including India, about the adverse reaction to foods. However because of lack of data in food allergy in India it is quite difficult to evaluate the allergenicty of GM food."[80]

Israel

"The overall prevalence of clinically relevant IgE-mediated food allergic reactions among these [Israeli] patients is estimated to be just over one percent. The most common food allergens were egg, cow's milk, and sesame. Anaphylaxis was the presenting symptom in eighteen percent including six sesame-induced cases. A history of other atopic diseases was reported in thirty-five percent of patients. In addition, twenty-eight percent had a history of atopy in first-degree family members...We found sesame to be a major cause of IgE-mediated food allergy in Israel. In fact, it is second only to cow's milk as a cause of anaphylaxis. We recommend that testing for food allergens be tailored to each community based on local experience and should include sesame in appropriate populations," per Pediatric Allergy and Clinical Immunology Unit, Israel.[81]

"Sesame seed allergy in Israel is as common as peanut allergy is in Europe and the U.S.," Wolf told The Jerusalem Post. "Here, the consumption of sesame seeds in its various forms is high, starting with six-month-old infants, because it is a very nutritional protein."[82]

Interestingly, "Camel's milk cures severe food allergies and rehabilitates the immune system in children, according to the results of a small study in Beersheba. Since it involved only eight children—all of whom recovered from their serious allergies after a short course of drinking the milk—the researchers have applied for approval for a much larger study to Soroka-University Medical Center...The parents were given frozen camel's milk from a hygienic source and were told to defrost rather than heat it because heat would destroy the protective immunoglobulins and proteins. Within twenty-four hours of their first 'dose,' all the children showed reduced symptoms, and after four days all symptoms of food allergies had disappeared, the authors reported. Some of those participating in the survey continued drinking camel's milk for a month. Their recovery was 'spectacular,' the researchers marveled."[83]

Italy

"An estimated six to eight percent of the Italian population has food allergies." Common food allergies: "Cow's milk, hen's egg, wheat, fish, tree-nut, and peanut. In Italy, E.U. regulations are followed. All ingredients are included on the label. The exceptions are composite products, where ingredients less than twenty-five percent of the product are not labeled)," per the Food Allergy and Anaphylaxis Network and Food Allergy Italia.[84]

Japan

"The recent increase of patients suffering from food allergy has become a social problem in Japan. A study by the Ministry of Health, Labor and Welfare (MHLW) reported that the Allergen labeling System under Food Sanitation Law was enacted on April 1, 2001. The Labeling System enables consumers to obtain information about the presence of allergenic ingredients in food and to avoid such food. Pre-packed processed food and food additives which contain following 'specified ingredients' are subject to this regulation. Five 'specified ingredients': egg, milk, and wheat (which cause food allergy with high frequency), as well as buckwheat and peanuts (which cause serious health hazards) are obliged to be labeled. Additionally, twenty ingredients: abalone, squid, salmon roe, shrimp/prawn, oranges, crab, kiwifruit, beef, tree nuts, salmon, mackerel, soybeans, chicken, pork, mushrooms, peaches, yams, apples, gelatin, and banana are recommended to be labeled. Food containing 'specified ingredients' must be labeled regardless of the quantity. 'May contain' type labeling without any rational foundation is forbidden. Food of concern is inspected according to ELISA (blood) tests at the initial screening step. Food samples that generate positive results with the ELISA tests are then sent for confirmatory testing by means of Western blotting/PCR tests plus the examination of manufacturing records," per Morinaga Institute of Biological Science, Inc.[85]

The Netherlands

"In the Netherlands, approximately 350,000 people suffer from food allergies." Anaphylaxis is believed to affect 12,000 persons. Common food allergies: "Peanut, milk, egg, wheat, tree nuts (almonds, hazelnut, cashew, walnut, etc.), soy, fish, shellfish, and sesame seed. The Netherlands follows labeling regulations set by the European Union (EU). Ingredients of flavorings are not required to be listed individually. Several foods do not have to list an ingredient statement. These can include single ingredient foods, such as fresh fruits and vegetables, and foods sold for immediate consumption. All ingredients must be listed. The exception is a composite ingredient, unless it constitutes more than twenty-five percent of the total product weight. The additives in this composite product, however, do have to be labeled regardless of weight. For example, if the slice of salami on a pizza *makes up less than twenty-five percent* of the finished product the ingredients of the salami would *not* have to be declared. The ingredients would just list 'salami.' In late 2001, the European Commission announced new plans to require the labeling of ingredients making up less than twenty-five percent of the final food product. If approved, this would affect all products sold in the European Union market. This proposal will effectively abolish the twenty-five percent rule described in the preceding paragraph. But the proposal has not yet been approved. Most major manufacturers and retailers have voluntarily agreed to ignore the twenty-five percent rule in which peanuts and nuts are concerned. They will always declare them. Some companies have extended this to other ingredients (e.g., milk, egg, sesame)," per the Food Allergy and Anaphylaxis Network and Nederlands Anafylaxis Netwerk.[86]

New Zealand

"Data is not available on the prevalence of food allergies." Common Food Allergies: "Eggs, wheat, soy, milk, peanuts, tree nuts, fish, and shellfish. These eight foods account for ninety percent of all food allergies. However, almost any food can cause an allergy. The Food Standards Australia New Zealand (FSANZ) regulates packaged labeling. Additives are listed by common name or according to their code number; for example, flavor enhancer (MSG) or flavor enhancer (621). Under the new ANZFA Food Standards Code (2002), wheat, gluten-containing cereals, crustacea, eggs, fish, milk, tree nuts, sesame seeds, peanuts, soy, and sulfites must be named on the ingredient list at all times without exception. The cutoff for all other component ingredients is now five percent. The use of class names (i.e., 'starch' or 'vegetable oil') has been restricted for the foods listed in the previous paragraph)," per the Food Allergy and Anaphylaxis Network and Allergy New Zealand.[87]

Russia, Estonia, Lithuania

"[A] self-reported food hypersensitivity in Sweden, Denmark, Estonia, Lithuania and Russia [was performed in which] patients with a history of food hypersensitivity completed a questionnaire and…skin-prick tests were performed. In Russia, Estonia, and Lithuania, citrus fruits, chocolate, honey, apple, hazelnut, strawberry, fish, tomato, egg, and milk were most often reported as causes of hypersensitivity. In Sweden and Denmark; birch pollen related foods, such as nuts, apple, pear, kiwi, stone fruits, and carrot were the most common causes. In all countries, children, more often than adults, had symptoms of allergic reaction to citrus fruits, tomato, strawberry, milk, egg, and fish…Severe symptoms were most common with fish, shellfish, nuts, and milk. Slight symptoms were most common with rice, coriander, poppy seed, lingonberry, corn, caraway, red currant, and fig."[88]

South Africa

"It is estimated that only between one and four percent of the general population suffers from a definite food allergy. Food allergy tends to be more common in children (up to six percent) than adults. In selected groups, such as children with eczema, the prevalence of food allergy may be as high as twenty-five percent. Foods which most often cause such reactions are peanut, milk, wheat, seafood, celiac (gluten), eggs, nuts, shellfish, citrus fruits and berries. Several foods have been shown to trigger migraine: chocolate, red wine, yeast extracts, hard cheeses, milk and eggs," per Allergy Society of South Africa.[89]

Spain

"Our results showed the principal foods involved in allergic reactions are: eggs, fish, and cow's milk. These are followed in frequency by fruits (peaches, hazelnuts and walnuts), legumes (lentils, peanuts and chick peas) and other vegetables (mainly sunflower seeds). The legumes demonstrated the highest degree of clinical cross-reactivity. Most patients with food allergy reacted to one or two foods (almost eighty-seven percent). Only thirteen percent of patients reacted to three or more foods, mostly to legumes and fruits. We found that food allergy begins most frequently in the first (forty-nine percent) and second (twenty percent) years of life. Allergy to proteins of cow's milk, egg, and fish begins predominantly before the second year, demonstrating a clear relationship with the introduction of these foods into the child's diet. Allergy to foods of vegetable origin (fruits, legumes and other vegetables) begins predominantly after the second year," per Immuno-allergy Laboratory, La Paz Children's Hospital, Madrid, Spain.[90]

United Kingdom

"According to the Anaphylaxis Campaign, statistics are hard to come by, but 1 in 100 children is believed to suffer severe allergic reactions to peanuts, tree nuts, or both. A small number are affected by other foods." Common Food Allergies: "Peanuts, tree nuts (almonds, hazelnuts, cashews, walnuts, etc.), sesame seeds, fish, shellfish, eggs, and milk. The U.K. follows labeling regulations set by the European Union (EU). Ingredients of flavorings are not required to be listed individually. Several foods do not have to list an ingredient statement. These can include single ingredient foods, such as fresh fruits and vegetables, and foods sold for immediate consumption. All ingredients must be listed. The exception is a composite ingredient, unless it constitutes more than twenty-five percent of the total product weight. The additives in this composite product, however, do have to be labeled regardless of weight. For example, if the slice of salami on a pizza makes up less than twenty-five percent of the finished product the ingredients of the salami would not have to be declared. The ingredients would just list 'salami.' In late 2001, the European Commission announced new plans to require the labeling of ingredients making up less than twenty-five percent of the final food product. If approved, this would affect all products sold in the European Union market. This proposal will effectively abolish the twenty-five percent rule described in the preceding paragraph. But the proposal has not yet been approved. Most major manufacturers and retailers have voluntarily agreed to ignore the twenty-five percent rule where peanuts and nuts are concerned. They will always declare them. Some companies have extended this to other ingredients (e.g., milk, egg, sesame)," per the Food Allergy and Anaphylaxis Network and Anaphylaxis Campaign.[91]

United States

In 2005, the number of people with food allergies in the U.S. was estimated at four percent or 11.4 million people,[92] Children have a higher rate of food allergies—between six to eight percent or about 1 in 13 children. Food-induced anaphylaxis is believed to cause 30,000 emergency room visits and between 150 and 200 deaths annually." Common Food Allergies: "Dairy, eggs, peanuts, tree nuts (almonds, hazelnuts, cashews, walnuts, etc.), fish, shellfish, soy, and wheat. In the United States, the Food and Drug Administration regulates packaged food. Ingredients must be noted on the label and are listed by name. Ingredients in food coloring, flavors, and spices are not required to be listed. Ingredients may appear on a label in technical or scientific terms. For example, casein is milk, albumen is egg. Products labeled as non-dairy may contain milk. Ingredients can sometimes change without warning)," per the Food Allergy and Anaphylaxis Network and Food Allergy & Anaphylaxis Network.[93]

West Africa, Ghana

"A study in rural and urban environments in Ghana is investigating the role of infections, particularly parasites, in the development of allergies to peanut, a food widely consumed in Ghana."[94] It appears that Ghana is one of the first countries in Africa (aside from South Africa) to begin its studies of food allergies. In collaboration with other countries, Ghana is beginning its research, "Complementary studies in Ghana, Western Siberia, India and China will allow us to gain insights into how different dietary patterns and exposure to microorganisms affect food allergies...To address one aspect of this, a small study is being undertaken in rural and urban environments in Ghana to investigate the role of infections, particularly parasites, in the development of allergies to peanut, a food widely consumed in Ghana."[95]

Part 2: The Solutions

In Part 1 of *Flourishing with Food Allergies*, the problem was discussed in a variety of ways. Specifically, we learned how food allergies affect many families all around us, but that we might not know it because we don't talk enough about it. There are probably people with whom you interact every day who have food allergies. Furthermore, food allergies do not just affect people in the United States. People all over the world have food allergies. It appears to me that the most common food allergies are to cow's milk, eggs, fish, shellfish and various legumes and nuts such as peanuts, walnuts and sesame seeds. I find it interesting to see the similarity and differences in food allergies from country to country.

We also reviewed the various reactions to foods during parents' stories which include vomiting, eczema and the most severe, anaphylactic shock—a sudden, severe allergic reaction characterized by a sharp drop in blood pressure, urticaria (hives), breathing difficulties...and which may be fatal if emergency treatment, including epinephrine injections, is not given immediately.[96] There may also be additional reactions through the delayed-antibody allergic reaction such as autism, ADHD and asthma where the symptoms of these disorders do not appear for several hours or days after eating the offending foods. Furthermore, the use of genetically modified foods, pesticides, hormones, and antibiotics may contribute to the recent increase in food allergies, especially in the small, sensitive bodies of our children. Additional attention, funding and research is needed to confirm these reactions.

In the next section various *solutions* are explored by way of interviews with doctors, teachers, a therapist and a father. Training, experience and beliefs differ with each interviewee, but there are common threads about what has worked well for each. None of these perspectives or ideas should be used in place of medical advice from your doctor for your child, but simply can serve as "food" for thought.

In addition to the interviews, research of allergen ingredients is provided as well as my experience with probiotics, the social aspects of handling food-filled social events, locating food-free activities for young children, and planning for travel and entering school.

To further aid parents in determining what is best for their child, it would be helpful to have more conclusive studies on the cause, testing and treatment for food allergies. For this purpose I have provided a sample letter which can by copied and mailed for the purpose of asking our federal government to allocate more funding for research of food allergies. This can be found in the conclusion of this book.

Perspectives

INTRODUCTION

I thought it would be valuable to interview several different types of medical doctors to show different viewpoints on similar questions. Traditional pediatricians, an allergist, and a naturopath were interviewed. Each was asked a similar set of questions, yet each interpreted the questions differently and had interesting opinions based upon his or her own experiences in practice. A psychotherapist was also interviewed to lend a perspective on the parent's emotional responses to food allergies in a young child.

Here are the questions that were asked:

- What is your educational background?

- How many years have you been in practice?

- Why did you choose your specialty?

- Have you seen the incidence of food allergies rise?

- Why do you think the incidence of food allergies has risen?

- Do you have any advice on the differences between traditional or naturopath allergists?

- What type of allergy testing do you recommend and why?

- How do you feel children are socially and emotionally affected?

- How do you feel parents are socially and emotionally affected?

- How do you believe food allergies affect parents and children who don't have food allergies?

- What advice can you give to parents of young children?

- Do you have any other perspectives, ideas or advice regarding food allergies in young children?

Finally, my husband's perspective is expressed on how to best accept and deal with food allergies from a father's point-of-view.

CHAPTER 32: ROMAN ALDER, M.D., PEDIATRICS

Dr. Roman Alder was originally a German citizen and moved to Romania in 1978 to carry out his pre-med studies. He returned to Berlin, Germany in 1982 to complete medical school and he graduated in 1986. He searched "high and low" from Scotland to Germany for the right training position and selected a clerkship position in the United States at Hurley Medical Center in Flint, Michigan, a public, non-profit, teaching medical center. He was then accepted into New York's Stony Brook University where he did his residency and graduated in 1991. Dr. Alder selected a practice in pediatrics because he wasn't interested in surgery and preferred the personal interaction with his patients. During his early years in practice, Dr. Alder accepted a position in a medically "underserved area" located in Alabama. He spent eight years helping this community and left only when it was no longer in great need of medical services.

Dr. Alder believes that while food allergy rates appear to be on the rise, recalling that peanut allergy has doubled from 1997 to 2002, he isn't convinced that all food allergies are rising at the reported rates. He believes that the public's awareness and the medical community's diagnoses of food allergies have increased, thus causing the numbers to appear higher. In other words, based upon his experience, it appears food allergies have probably been around for a long time in great numbers, but in the past may have not been diagnosed as such. Furthermore, Dr. Alder is not convinced that food allergies contribute to ADHD or autism.

Dr. Alder states that medical perspectives can differ in diagnoses and treatment. The allopathic physician, one who is trained in traditional non-homeopathic, non-naturopathic medicine, has a perspective that is often in contrast to the naturopathic physician. Dr. Alder's perspectives are based on the allopathic training that he received during his medical studies and admits he is not well versed in naturopathic techniques or remedies. With respect to food allergies, he believes both camps will agree that avoidance of the allergy producing food is the best course of action.

Based upon his experience and research, Dr. Alder believes that a person can be sensitized to foods in utero. If the mother has or had a sensitivity when younger, and if she eats those foods to which she was allergic while she is pregnant, then the baby can become sensitized to the food even before birth. He would advise a pregnant mother-to-be to avoid eating foods to which she or her family history has shown a sensitivity or allergy. Dr. Alder further points out the disagreement in the medical community about these recommendations because there is no conclusive evidence or studies. After all, it is not easy to carry out studies on people because it is so challenging and life changing to alter one's diet so completely that most people are not willing to do it for the sake of science. He further explains that medical viewpoints are unclear about issues such as when it is best to introduce solid foods to babies. Some advise to give solid foods as early as three months, while others advise waiting until between one and two years of age. Dr. Alder believes that the best age would be between three to six months, but again to avoid foods to which there is a family history of allergies.

He recalls that several years of practice passed before he came to this realization of how hard it is for families to eliminate a food or foods from their diets. He describes, "Once it clicked for me, I realized the dramatic changes and challenges to the parent when the diagnosis of a food allergy is made." When a child exhibits a food allergy, Dr. Alder gives advice with caution because he has learned how drastic the diagnosis of a food allergy can be and its impact on a family's life. For example, he states, "If a child is allergic to wheat, dairy and nuts then simply sitting at a Thanksgiving dinner table can be a stress provoking situation."

Furthermore, he states, "Taking the child to an allergy specialist is a must if the food allergies are serious enough to cause anaphylaxis. These types of food allergies are beyond the scope of a general practitioner who can perform certain allergy tests like the newer Immunocap blood test, found to be ninety percent accurate in adults, but general practitioners cannot perform the more detailed skin prick and RAST blood tests."

Dr. Alder believes that the best way to handle food allergies, aside from food avoidance, is to be assertive and proactive. He points out that living in the United States can support this approach. He states, "Parents should educate themselves and should not rely too heavily on their physicians. Getting a second or third medical opinion, reading books and articles on the Internet is an excellent way to become an expert on the issue."

Dr. Alder further believes, "Unless a person personally has to deal with severe anaphylaxis risk food allergies for himself or herself or a family member, it is extremely difficult, if not impossible, to understand and fully grasp the issue. In other words, people who have no true food allergies cannot understand what it is like to deal with them. Because food allergies can be so difficult to handle, some hospitals have created coping classes and camps for families of food allergic people."

There is an important positive characteristic that can emerge from this situation. Dr. Alder points out, "When a child has food allergies, he or she is forced to become disciplined and assertive in order to survive. He cannot eat certain foods so must ask what is in foods before eating." He further believes, "These qualities of discipline and assertiveness can serve the child well when he is an adult in the professional world. He is likely to be more successful."

CHAPTER 33: JOSEF BURTON, M.D., PEDIATRICS

Dr. Josef Burton received two bachelor degrees, a B.A. from University of Rochester in history and a B.S. from Syracuse University in biology. He then received his medical degree from Dalhousie University in Nova Scotia, Canada. He elected a specialty in pediatrics because he liked working with children since they are just starting their lives and are free from chronic illnesses. Dr. Burton earned a Master of Science degree from Ohio State University where he remained to teach Clinical Pediatrics for three years. He has practiced pediatric medicine for thirty-five years in New York, Massachusetts and Connecticut.

Dr. Burton believes that in recent years allergies have increased. He states, "Both environmental and food allergies have increased, especially for those with a family history of allergies and a higher level of sensitivity to our environment. Things that heighten sensitivities in today's marketplace include sunscreens, fabric softeners, antibiotics, hormones and processing ingredients to extend the shelf life of foods." He explains, "Fabric sheets that we use to soften our clothing in the dryer are a big irritant to the skin. The softener chemical goes all over the clothing, inside and out, and leaves a film that touches our skin for hours while we wear our clothes and sleep in our bed. This film is a chemical that can irritate many children's skin causing a rash. Even if there is no rash, the chemical still enters the child's body through the skin, adding one more toxin to the child's system that can cause allergic symptoms."

Dr. Burton says, "Other chemicals entering the body such as perfumes in detergents and soaps, and dyes in these products and our foods can cause an allergic reaction. If a child has a propensity to develop food allergies, then these toxins accumulate in the child's body and if too many of them are present on a given day or in general, then the child will begin to exhibit severe allergies to the environment and to foods. Furthermore, a history of food allergies in the family, a mother's and a father's sensitivity to a food can increase the likelihood of developing food allergies. Any food which has caused a problem in a family, like nuts or shellfish, may be a problem to the child."

Dr. Burton describes his two theories of allergies, "First there is the *Camel Effect*. For instance, if a child consumes milk, soy, fish and chicken in a single day, all to which the child is sensitive, then on that day the child might show a reaction by developing hives, for instance. But on a different day, if the child has only two or three of those offending foods, then the child might not exhibit a reaction. Similarly, there is the *Amount Effect*. For example, if a child can only handle a limited amount of dairy and if the child has too much of it in a single day, such as a glass of milk, a yogurt, and an ice cream cone, then he might develop a reaction." When a child's body is inundated with just cow's milk or just soy milk, the child develops a reaction. He states, "It isn't surprising that soy is the second most common allergen in children because if they aren't drinking cow's milk, they're drinking soy milk."

Dr. Burton states that the Camel Effect and Amount Effect have been more apparent in recent years because of all of the additional chemicals used in our foods now as compared to when we and our parents were growing up. For example, "Chickens are now treated with estrogen hormones to make the chicken grow larger and plumper. When our young girls eat chicken, their breasts start developing abnormally early. I advise mothers to stop feeding chicken to their young daughters when they complain of this problem. Most mothers report that eliminating chicken stops the problem from continuing." Similarly, Dr. Burton explains, "Cows are pumped up with antibiotics and hormones so it is not surprising that the most common childhood allergy is to cow's milk. Why are we drinking cow's milk? Cow's milk is for cows, not people. Cows have four stomachs, we have one."

The solution to developing allergies is to expose the child to a wide variety of foods and practice food rotation. A child can begin eating solid foods between four and six months, and maybe even earlier according to

Dr. Burton. He recommends starting with cereals, then vegetables, since they are bitter and children will like them less than other foods. He continues, "Then try fruits then proteins such as chicken, turkey, fish and meat. Further, parents need to make a serious effort to increase the variety of the foods that they eat themselves. Just because parents haven't tried lima beans, string beans or carrots in twenty years, doesn't mean that they shouldn't try them again." Dr. Burton recalls, "Many mothers look at me funny when I tell them this and they say, 'We don't eat fish' (for example). Parents need to eat these foods as well. Children mimic their parents, so if a parent will not eat fish, then the child won't either."

Food rotation will happen naturally if the child eats with his or her family. "A common mistake that parents make," explains Dr. Burton, "is that they will give their child his or her favorite food, just to get them to eat something. For instance, if the child likes chicken nuggets, then even though the parents are having meatloaf or ham for dinner with vegetables and brown rice, the child will be served chicken nuggets and French fries. Then, the next night the same thing happens because the child knows he can get the chicken nuggets if he refuses the other foods." Dr. Burton says, "Parents should make one meal for the entire family. Then if a child refuses to eat it, he can go a bit hungry. He'll make up for it the next day. Children won't starve themselves. Serving one meal is better for the child because it teaches him to eat what the family eats and exposes him to more foods. It is better for the child in the long run."

He continues, "Another problem with today's foods are the quick and easy meals that many parents like to buy and serve, rather than taking the time to cook a meal from scratch. Parents complain that they are too busy to cook. But foods that are prepared ahead of time are heavily processed. Our labeling laws are improving, but they need to improve more to show all the ingredients used in processing foods." Dr. Burton explains, "There are active ingredients and inert ingredients in our foods. Inert ingredients may remain in foods when processing is done. Terms like food stabilizer or thickener are used but the ingredients aren't listed on the label—the laws don't require manufacturers to list all the chemicals that are used in food processing—food coloring, eggs, and red dyes can be another source of allergies. A child can be allergic to hidden ingredients in the food." He suggests that parents try to eat foods that are natural and good for the human body, such as fish, liver (a good source of iron), ham, pork, and lamb along with organic fresh fruits, vegetables, and natural grains like brown rice.

Dr. Burton states, "Back when we were kids and our parents were kids, our foods weren't radiated, cloned or genetically modified. The animals we ate weren't treated with antibiotics or hormones. Overexposure to antibiotics in our meat causes our own bodies to be overexposed thereby causing an allergy to antibiotics as well as antibiotic resistant bacteria to develop. Pesticides probably contribute to food allergies and even worse to cancer."

Dr. Burton believes, "The best way to ascertain whether a child has food allergies is talk to the mother or father, whoever is the primary caretaker. If the primary caretaker is prudent and aware, then she knows that the child reacts after eating certain foods. Further, she knows the reaction goes away once the child stops eating the offending food. The mother *can* accurately assess the child's reactions *if* she is conscientious." Dr. Burton prefers to listen to the mother because he feels that invasive testing, like skin prick and blood testing, should be avoided on children under two. Kinesiology testing is an alternative if it can be accurately done on a child that young. But again, the mother is often the best source of information.

Dr. Burton states, "For treatments of food allergies, avoidance of the offending foods is the key, along with serving a variety of organic, non-ready-made foods." He is wary of supplements and elixirs because they would not naturally be found in the body through the consumption of food. Any substance that doesn't come naturally into the body by way of food, but prepared by doctors or scientists, can be considered a medication. The strength of any medication can be too much for a child and cause a new problem. For instance, he explains, "Too much vitamin A can cause headaches. Too much vitamin D can lead to poisoning. It is better to treat a child with celiac disease by avoiding all gluten foods."

Dr. Burton believes that children are affected in many ways by the foods we eat and the air we breathe. He explains, "Reactions can be both visible and invisible. We can see rashes and hives, but there are reactions that are not as easy to identify such as grumpiness and irritability. If a child's tongue or lips can swell, why can't his brain swell too? Offending foods probably make our internal organs swell at times that can make it difficult or nearly impossible for a child to do the things we expect, such as sit and study or act the way we expect him to act." He believes that people need to be more educated—it alleviates anger. On a positive note, Dr. Burton believes that over the past five years or so, children, parents, teachers, and chefs are becoming more aware and accepting of food allergies.

CHAPTER 34: PAMELA KWITTKEN, M.D., ALLERGIST

Dr. Pamela Kwittken graduated in 1982 from the University of Pennsylvania with a major in biomedical anthropology and minor in chemistry. She attended Sackler School of Medicine in Israel for which she learned to speak Hebrew. She graduated in 1987 from medical school and entered a residency program at Bellevue Hospital/NYC Medical Center until 1990. She did a fellowship at Children's Hospital in Pennsylvania from 1990 to 1992 and accepted a position at New York University Medical Center under a Grant for Pediatric Allergists Program for Inner City Children from 1992 to 1994. She then worked at a health center and moved into private practice eventually opening her own practice seven years ago.

During her training, she worked with allergists and pediatric doctors in the areas of immunology and oncology (cancer). She found it too distressing to watch the children suffering from leukemia, without the advances in care that are available today, to pursue that line of medicine. In the field of immunology, she experienced an outbreak in latex allergies and she treated many children with asthma. She now considers that some of those children may have been suffering from food allergies as well. Dr. Kwittken reports, "I have seen the incidence of food allergies rise over the past twenty years. Then food allergies—primary egg, peanut, and soy—appeared to affect children and adults equally, but today the number of children with food allergies far outnumbers that of adults and the number of foods to which children are allergic has grown as well."

Dr. Kwittken believes there are many possible reasons for the increase in food allergies in today's children. She advises, "One reason for an increase in the food allergies is because we are able to recognize it better. In the past we probably treated many allergy sufferers with asthma medication. Now we consider the symptoms of rash and seizures to be those of a food allergy. Another reason for the increase is because we are eating highly processed foods. Some studies show that the food additives in many foods make children and adults, eat beyond their point of normal satiety, e.g., the brain signaling the body that enough caloric intake has been received. Also I would postulate that perhaps these additives may play a role in food allergies, an area as yet unexplored. Another study demonstrates that babies can absorb the saliva from a kiss on their cheek which can increase their exposure to chemicals and allergens from an adult's lips. Additionally, many babies suffer from acid reflux, normally a condition of overweight adults, but in children this condition decreases the protective barrier to the gut, possibly making it less able to digest some proteins in foods, thereby, causing food allergies. Another theory is the 'tight house syndrome' that postulates that babies inhale cooked food allergens that are in the air of the home, thereby, irritating their immune systems and triggering food allergies."

With all of these relatively new onslaughts to a child's body, the immune system is reacting, or overreacting. Dr. Kwittken recommends that children who are exhibiting allergic symptoms (such as hives, rash, and circles under the eyes) undergo a blood test for allergies. She states, "I used to administer skin prick tests first, as was common by most allergists, but because of the risk of severe allergic reaction, there are cases in which blood tests are recommended instead. So for safety, if it is possible to draw blood from a baby, I will use the blood test. It is difficult to take blood from a two-month-old, but at one or two years it is possible with a skilled nurse. I don't think it is any more traumatic to stick a child with a needle to draw blood than it is to stick a child with several sets of skin prick testing needles. If the blood test comes back negative, then the skin prick test can be used to double check for an allergic response. Sometimes the skin prick test can come back negative, even though the child exhibits a reaction to the actual food. This is because the allergen sample used for the test can be too pure and sterile. One way around this is to use the real food, like a strawberry, rather than the prepared strawberry sample. Additionally, there is a new kind of test being used in Europe called a patch test. The patch is left on the skin for three days and can test for delayed food reactions. This test is not yet standardized and the allergen sample used can vary widely. A final complicating factor is that in addition to false negatives, some foods can exhibit a false positive (irritant) reaction so therefore must be interpreted by a skilled clinician."

Dr. Kwittken continues, "Once the food allergies are identified, whether the doctor is a traditional allergist or a naturopath allergist, almost all will agree that elimination of the offending food is the best route to take. Many traditional allergists recommend a rotation diet to help prevent additional food allergies from developing. Specifically, rotating foods over seven days will help to prevent malnutrition and hold off additional allergies from too much of one food. The naturopath might also supplement a child with antioxidants to help the child's body heal itself. There is a chance of outgrowing some food allergies. Specifically the best chance is for outgrowing allergies to dairy and egg. About twenty percent outgrow peanut, six percent outgrow tree nut, but virtually none outgrow seafood allergies."

Dr. Kwittken believes, "Parents can best handle food allergies in their child by not being overprotective but instead taking a more logical mindset by monitoring their child's diet through carefully reading labels. It is actually easier to monitor a younger child's diet as compared to an adolescent's diet. Once the child becomes a teenager, he or she becomes rebellious and prone to peer-pressure. For instance, a teenager may have a boyfriend or girlfriend whom he or she kisses or otherwise become intimate. Tests have been done that show that peanut remains in the saliva for hours, even after brushing teeth. Further, teenagers don't want to be bothered with carrying EpiPens®. Then once the teenager is in college, he is normally forced to join and pay for the meal plan. But it can be difficult, if not dangerous for those who have food allergies to eat in the cafeteria because many foods become aerosolized and otherwise contaminated through cooking oils and surfaces."

"With respect to youngsters just entering school, there are a few options," reports Dr. Kwittken. "In a few other states, the governor has mandated that children with food allergies shall be protected through an 'Act Concerning Food Allergies and the Prevention of Life-Threatening Incidents in School,' which was enacted by the Senate and House of Representatives. This act provides a sample action plan which can be used to explain the food allergies and response needed to teachers, nurses and other school officials without going to the extent of a 504 Disability Plan. This new mandate has greatly improved the attitude of schools in caring for children with food allergies. Previously the attitude was often, 'If a child has food allergies, then he or she should be home schooled.' Several years ago, at parties or other social events, parents would ask me if I thought it was an overreaction not to allow certain foods in the classroom. I always surprised and disappointed them by telling them that they were wrong and the foods should be eliminated for the sake of the allergic child," she explains.

"But now, people are more understanding and educated about food allergies," she believes. "Home schooling can be more socially isolating than dealing with food allergies in the regular school system. Much of the flexibility still depends upon the school itself. Some schools, especially bigger ones, are less flexible about allowing children to carry EpiPen® Jrs. and asthma inhalers than smaller schools. On a positive note, I know a smaller school where the nurse is so caring that she will bake allergen-free cupcakes for parties for the entire class for the sake of the food allergic child."

"One area of concern that remains," reports Dr. Kwittken, "is the school bus. The bussing is not normally part of the school, it is a separate entity. The bus drivers are not trained on how to use an EpiPen® Jrs. and even though children are not supposed to eat on the bus, some do. I have trained first graders on how to self-administer the EpiPen® Jr. so that they are able to bring it onto the bus. Of course, it depends upon the intelligence and maturity of the child—not all first graders might be capable of this responsibility. But because many young children want to ride the school bus, it is an option that can work."

In summary, Dr. Kwittken says, "Over the years the media has helped to educate all parents. This has made everyone more willing to help children with food allergies. Parents of food allergic children might be anxious on the one hand, but on the other hand, they are more aware parents. They should realize that although the food allergy might be a lifelong condition, it need not be a social disability. While the child is young, it is important to monitor his food by reading labels carefully to eliminate all allergens from his diet. Another idea is to use probiotics, although studies have only proven that probiotics help *prevent* food allergies, not *cure* existing food allergies. Since there are no side effects, it is worth a try under the supervision of a child's pediatrician. Some of the other remedies in research, such as Chinese herbal medications, are not recommended because they can be very toxic to the liver. Although some allergists disagree, I advise my patients to avoid giving children peanuts and tree nuts until at least two to three years of age. I also recommend feeding children organic foods, primarily because organic foods are better for the child, but also because it is easier to identify allergens when there are fewer ingredients in the food."

I would encourage parents to take their child to an allergist if they suspect food allergies are causing the symptoms in their child. At best, if the results are negative, then food allergies can be ruled out as the cause. Otherwise, if food allergies are to be found the culprit, then a food elimination diet can be started with confidence.

CHAPTER 35: JOSH BERRY, N.D., NATUROPATH

Dr. Josh Berry was brought up in Oregon under the care of a naturopath physician. In high school, he knew he wanted to be a doctor and considered pediatric surgery but decided on naturopath medicine based upon his own positive experience. He attended the University of Oregon for his undergraduate studies. In 1998, he graduated from the National College of Natural Medicine, a naturopathic school and classical Chinese medicine school, located in Portland, Oregon. Dr. Berry opened a practice in Eugene, Oregon but eventually moved across the country to teach pediatrics, clinical diagnosis and ear, nose and throat medicine at the University of Bridgeport in Connecticut between 2000 and 2003. He joined and eventually took over a practice in Connecticut eight years ago.

Dr. Berry states that naturopath doctors, whose suffix is N.D. (instead of the M.D. normally following a traditional medical doctor's name), are fully trained as doctors and depending on the state in which they practice, they can be licensed to prescribe pharmaceutical medications and perform surgery just as their traditional counterparts. In addition to these skills, naturopath doctors are also trained in homeopathy, as are chiropractors. This training takes place during their four year medical school training by taking additional credits each semester. The average number of credits carried by a naturopath student is eighteen to twenty-four, whereas most other students take between sixteen to eighteen credits.

Dr. Berry explains, "My naturopath practice has always focused on food allergies. There is a big difference between a food allergy and intolerance. If there is an IgE antibody in the body, generated by the body's immune system, then a true food allergy exists. In contrast, food intolerances are sensitivities to foods which might cause a stomachache or other symptom but the immune antibodies are not involved." Dr. Berry states that although the incidence of food allergies has been reported to increase in recent years, much of the increase may be due to an increased awareness and diagnoses of food allergies. In the past, the food allergies might have been incorrectly diagnosed as something else. Although this phenomenon might be occurring, Dr. Berry does agree that more and more infants and young children are experiencing true allergic reactions to foods.

Dr. Berry points out that the possible causes of food allergies are probably found in the foods we eat today as compared to when he was a child. For instance, children in today's schools often bring pre-packaged lunches, such as cheese and crackers in a ready made plate covered in plastic that can sit on the shelf for a long time. He states, "When we were kids, we would eat a sandwich and some carrot and celery sticks or an apple on the side." He further points out that the cafeterias in the schools rarely make food from scratch. Instead, they purchase pre-packaged ready-made foods filled with preservatives, then serve them to our children. Furthermore, the foods that we are purchasing from grocery stores are loaded with chemicals, pesticides, soil preparations and many foods are radiated and genetically modified.

He explains, "There is a lack of studies on food allergies in the United States." He points out that our capitalistic society has a tendency to invest in products that can be advertised and purchased by the public, thereby making a profit for a company. In other words, "Why would a company want to pay for a study that doesn't benefit them financially?" The unfortunate consequence of our capitalistic oriented country is the loss of the goal of being healthy and eating well. Not many groups will promote eating healthy foods if it doesn't directly impact their profits. Even worse, many companies sell their products as being healthy, whether or not they really are healthy.

"The fact is," according to Dr. Berry, "that food allergies exist. Many of my patients come from traditional medical doctors and are told that their ailments are not caused by something they are eating, when in fact, food is the cause." Dr. Berry investigates his patients' reactions to foods using a variety of tests. Often the first test used is called Applied Kinesiology. He uses this type of testing often with children because it is non-invasive and can help identify food sensitivities. Once a set of sensitivities is identified, the patient's diet can be revised to eliminate problem foods. After a few weeks on that revised diet the symptoms, such as hives or eczema, go away and the results of the test are confirmed. Other times, another test is needed. In those cases, Dr. Berry will call for a RAST blood test which tests for the presence of IgE antibodies. Although this test is fairly accurate, problems include locating delayed antibody reactions as with locating an IgG antibody which might not be created by the body for a day or so after eating a food. Further, the RAST test is less accurate in a child younger than two. Another test that Dr. Berry might call for is the Cell to Cell Interaction test. In this test, the patient's blood is taken and tested in a lab by exposing it to various foods in a petri dish. Still other options for testing might include Electro Acupuncture according to Voll (EAV) test, which is a way to determine energetically unbalanced points in a patient's body.

Once the results are in hand from the testing, Dr. Berry will recommend which foods should be removed from the diet for two months. During that time, he will provide tinctures and natural supplements to rebuild the body's immune system and reduce inflammation. A tincture is a mixture of herbal medicines to treat colds, asthma, congestion and infections. Supplements might include Acidophilus, a probiotic used to rebuild the digestive system by healing the intestinal lining. Another example of a supplement might be Quercetin a substance found in yellow onions that has anti-inflammatory effects. The supplements prescribed by naturopaths are stronger than those that can be purchased off-the-shelf at health food and grocery stores.

Once the patient has been taking the supplements for about two months, Dr. Berry will decide whether to do a challenge test on the offending foods. Usually the symptoms will have disappeared, such as eczema or hives, over this period of time. Further, the parent is often anxious to see if there is improvement. If the test of eating the offending food brings back the symptoms, then a longer treatment is needed. Sometimes mild sensitivities are healed after only a few months.

Dr. Berry believes that food allergies can impact a child's social and emotional well being. He states, "Much of the impact depends upon the child's own emotional sensitivity. Some children are simply more sensitive than other children. I don't want a child to have a negative self-esteem or an eating disorder so I am careful about the words that I use to explain the food allergies. I make sure to tell a child that a lot of people have food allergies and that it is part of life." Dr. Berry advises parents not to make the child feel different and to focus on the foods that he can eat. He admits, "Food allergies can be difficult when kids want to eat pizza with their friends."

Dr. Berry feels, "People who do not have food allergies don't really understand what it means to avoid foods completely. It just isn't on their radar. But when parents start to host play dates with food allergic children, they start to pay attention. They don't want anything to go wrong." He thinks, "There are two kinds of people: There are the people who just don't really pay attention. Then there are the people who overreact, out of fear. Often school personnel fall into this latter category." Dr. Berry advises, "Parents of young children with food allergies need to reach out. Don't be afraid to share what is going on in your situation. It will be much easier if you share with friends. There are more people than you might realize who are in the same situation."

CHAPTER 36: K. DAVID SCHULTZ, PH.D., ABPP, LICENSED CLINICAL PSYCHOLOGIST

Dr. David Schultz enjoyed talking with people ever since he was a youngster. He found it fascinating to discover why people did the things they did and wanted to help people, especially whenever he noticed that they might be making a decision that would affect their lives. After receiving his B.A. degree from the University of Michigan in 1971, he earned a Masters of Science degree in 1973 and Ph.D. in 1976 from Yale University. During his thirty year career, Dr. Schultz worked as instructor, psychologist (providing therapeutic services), psychotherapist (treating mental disorders) and Director of Psychological Services. He has been recognized numerous times in Who's Who publications and contributed to numerous written studies. Currently he works in private practice, serves on the adjunct professional staff at several hospitals, and is a lecturer at Yale University School of Medicine.

Dr. Schultz believes that food allergies may have increased in recent years based upon changes in the farming practices in the United States and the developed world, and even more so since worldwide trade has exponentially increased. "For instance," he recalls, "When I grew up in the Midwest in farm country, the produce and livestock were in general raised in a more natural, holistic, and healthy manner. For example, there were more small farms that practiced crop rotation which enriched the soil naturally thus making the foods generally more nutritious."

In today's farming practices, many small farms are gone and have instead been replaced by a few major agricultural businesses utilizing primarily inorganic fertilizers and monoculture. He believes that recent trends to increase yields dramatically have lead to the unintended consequence that many foods may have rapidly deteriorated in quality during the late 1980s and 1990s. He postulates that while new technologies, like genetically modified foods, might help with some aspects of our food supply, there may likely be unintended consequences which may remain unidentified and therefore underreported for an extended period of time, suggesting perhaps that one such consequence may be reflected in recent trends toward increased food sensitivities and allergies.

It is likely to take extended periods of time and ultimately may be difficult to prove that some food sensitivities and allergies are a consequence of our deteriorated food supply. He says, "The predominant approach in current scientific research in a number of fields appears to focus on demonstrating with certainty that something leads to something else, for most if not all cases." Dr. Schultz explains, "Some scientists appear to be seeking simple causative relationships applicable to the population in general. In other words, they tend to minimize what appear to be individual anomalies while emphasizing black and white answers applicable to larger groups of people."

But he continues, "Individuals are different, fundamentally unique, and thus have different sensitivities, so it is not easy to make these conclusions across the board. For instance, some children are more sensitive than others. Could the antibiotics in the milk cause these sensitive children to develop sensitivities or become allergic to some antibiotics and/or become antibiotic resistant more readily?"

Dr. Schultz further points to studies that show ADHD symptomatology can be exacerbated by lifestyle choices, diet, and even some food additives. Also, waiting to establish conclusive scientific proof of these possibilities is not only difficult but may neglect focusing on the fact that most people prefer to be viewed as individuals while not wanting to be treated in a trial and error fashion as if they were guinea pigs. Because individual differences may often override group trends, it is difficult to find solid relevant scientific studies and conclusions on specific food sensitivities and allergies.

In addition to difficulties in researching food allergies, the every day issues can be difficult for parents and children as well. For instance, Dr. Schultz points out how important the relationship between a doctor and patient can be. He states, "Whether the doctor is a traditional medical doctor or a naturopath doctor, the important factor is that the practitioner pays attention to the particular sensitivities of the child and what might cause allergies for him or her." Depending upon the situation, he states, "A more natural remedy might be in order such as removing metals and yeast from an autistic child's diet to improve the behavior. In addition to the child's sensitivities, the parent's level of acceptance must be taken into account. What kinds of treatment are the parents open to? Are they willing to consider the potential benefit of a natural remedy, complementary or alternative treatments, and if so, to what extent? For instance, are they open to exploring the introduction of graduated life style changes, an elimination diet, particular supplements, or even such seemingly irrelevant interventions as music, art, meditation, yoga, eurhythmy, or acupuncture?"

Another important factor in the doctor-patient relationship involves the nature and extent of communication. Dr. Schultz recommends that parents ask themselves, "Do I feel that I am being listened to? Do I feel that I am being respected? If I ask a question to which the doctor doesn't know the answer, does he acknowledge that, offer to research it and get back to me?" In contrast, if we feel that the doctor's attitude displays one of "I am the boss" thereby making us feel unimportant or disrespected, then that particular doctor may not be a good match. In addition to the importance of the relationship between the doctor and the patient, Dr. Schultz believes, "Modern human beings need to be advocates for themselves and their children. They need to read and become informed to help make decisions about what is best for their own particular situations."

Parents of food allergic children have a difficult situation, Dr. Schultz explains. Parents need to be sensitive to their child's ability to handle both physical and emotional overload. For instance, when a baby is developmentally ready to drink juice or other foods, most pediatricians advise parents to introduce to the child's diet only very small amounts of a single new food or juice and be watchful for any reactions.

Adding a new food too quickly or giving too much of a single food can overload a child's system causing a sensitivity or perhaps even contributing to the possibility of developing an allergy.

The overload may also occur on an emotional level. "Both parent and child can become extraordinarily frightened by a child's allergic reaction. For instance, when a child consumes a food which causes a symptom of difficulty breathing, it is terrifying," he explains, "It is important for parents to try to control their own emotions. If parents overreact or remain visibly panic stricken, it may make a potentially lifethreatening situation even worse."

Handling both the allergy situation and the fear it creates in a controlled way can take a huge toll on parents. Dr. Schultz finds, "Parents may often become hyper-vigilant and emotionally on edge because they must be extremely careful when taking their child into new environments. If they are not, the consequences can be severe, even lifethreatening. When friends, family members and others don't support parents' realistic concerns, then it makes it even more difficult for the parents to provide for their children's safety. Therefore, it becomes essential for doctors and other health care providers to pay significant attention to the parents *in addition* to the child. Better providers will listen to a parent's fears and some practitioners may even provide parent and family support groups for children with allergies as well as those with other potentially more serious medical concerns."

"While parents need to find support for themselves, they must also be a support system for their food-sensitive or food-allergic child," Dr. Schultz points out. "Living with food allergies can be challenging, so children need a strong support system. For instance, in school a child may have to sit at a peanut-free table for lunch. Other children may show a lack of empathy, since they often haven't thought about what it can feel like to have food allergies," Dr. Schultz explains. "Schools and parents may help by explaining things to all of the children in a way that is understandable to them. For instance, a parent or teacher might create a story or fairy tale that explains food allergies and what it feels like to have an allergic reaction. Further, the story line could provide examples of a socially responsible response to an allergic reaction. Even asking questions such as, 'What would it feel like if you couldn't breathe?' These questions can cause kids to imagine and really realize how terrible and frightening it would be. Even though everyone is different, we are also all the same in certain ways: Everyone needs to be able to breath. In this way, other children can learn to understand and empathize with what a food allergic child might feel like," he points out.

Dr. Schultz further explains, "Real life situations in our public schools have rapidly become extraordinarily complicated. Some school administrators and parent teacher organizations (PTOs) may make overly simplistic, 'zero-tolerance' decisions that have the unintended consequence of not working for all situations, often becoming unfair and even detrimental to particular children and families. Everyone, including administrators, parents and teachers, needs to become involved in order to arrive at socially-conscious solutions which maintain the safety as well as the emotional well-being of a food allergic child and his or her classmates."

"By having a comprehensive intervention arrived at through collaborative dialogue, some of the responsibility will be lifted from teachers, thereby, allowing them to be more productive in teaching children. Parents whose children don't have food allergies might not be as supportive as desired by others. Their lack of support may be the result of an oversimplified, incomplete understanding of food sensitivities and allergies," states Dr. Schultz. He recommends that people share their experience and learn with others in a collaborative manner so that social networks will function more effectively for everyone, while maintaining the goal of safety first.

On a positive note, Dr. Schultz believes, "A challenge can make a person stronger." This truism can be applied to both the parent and the child. Challenges can be faced with the assistance of other people through networking and self-help groups. Human beings need to be more self-aware, self-conscious and open to learning. There are a lot of excellent resources in a variety of forms, ranging from the Internet to local natural food stores, farmers' markets and community supported agriculture. He has seen the interest in local farmers' markets and the resulting growth of these markets as one indication of the increased awareness of modern consumers. Some people are now recognizing the importance of buying and eating organic foods from local farms, especially in light of the worldwide exponential increase in food sensitivities and allergies.

CHAPTER 37: MY HUSBAND'S PERSPECTIVE

In my life before children, I worked in the fields of law and computer science. I studied pre-law courses at UCLA and worked as a paralegal and office manager of a law office in Los Angeles. One of my responsibilities was to manage the computer systems, which I found interesting. As a result of this interest, I decided to take an engineering and business program in computer science at UCLA. This led to my current career in information technology.

After about ten years of marriage, my wife and I decided to have children. When my first son was about five months my wife gave him milk-based formula. He broke out in hives. This happened on the second try as well. After that, my wife spoke with a friend who hit the nail on the head and advised us that she believed our son was allergic to dairy. She was not afraid to tell us her opinion in a very straightforward manner which we greatly appreciated. My wife then called the doctor to discuss the matter and he told her to try once more. My wife declined to try the milk-based formula again. She began to mitigate risk by using a soy-based formula instead. While we were aware of the dairy allergy, we did not yet realize its full implications.

In fact, we were only slightly sensitized to allergies at first. At one point our son bit into a package of cheese and barely broke the plastic. He had a violent coughing attack that lasted for one minute or so. My wife was just about to panic when it stopped. Additionally, he developed a chronic cough—a constant hacking when playing. Evening after evening, I'd worry as my son coughed while we played just before bedtime. Of course, our cat was part of the action and I began to suspect that he might be allergic to her. As a result, we had him tested at age one for a variety of allergens. But we did not test our son for dairy because the allergist was sure he was allergic to dairy due to the hives after drinking the formula. The results showed he was allergic to chicken, egg, and the cat. The allergist recommended that we let the cat go, so that our son would not develop asthma. Although this was very hard for me, we did let the cat go and my son's coughing subsided. A year later, when our son was two, we had him re-tested for dairy and the results were quite high. I felt rather downhearted by it all.

In retrospect, I think I had a typical set of reactions when I learned of our first son's food allergies. In the past, I have had occasion to read about the "grief cycle," and I have found that the process of coping with food allergies is very much like the grief cycle. Specifically, the Kübler-Ross Grief Cycle has been characterized as follows:

> *Shock:* Initial paralysis at hearing the bad news.
> *Denial:* Trying to avoid the inevitable.
> *Anger:* Frustrated outpouring of bottled-up emotion.
> *Bargaining:* Seeking in vain for a way out.
> *Depression:* Final realization of the inevitable.
> *Testing:* Seeking realistic solutions.
> *Acceptance:* Finally finding the way forward.

This cycle is exactly the set of stages that I went through in dealing with my son's allergies. I passed from shock into denial quite quickly as most people do. I believe I lingered in the denial stage for some time. For instance, I actually gave my son a sour cream and onion potato chip. My response to my wife when she said this was not good was, "Oh, it's just a little bit." I am ashamed of that incident, because it is that kind of lack of understanding of the problem in others that today tends to make me revisit the anger and frustration stages. Food allergies are an important situation in which to minimize denial.

In the anger stage, I was not so much angry at anything or anybody in particular. At that point, I directed the anger or frustration towards getting angry at the problem itself. This is often how I get things done. I often demonize a problem then go after it. In other words, I use the anger phase to motivate myself.

The anger motivated me to research food allergies. Once I realized the seriousness of food allergies, I believe I entered the bargaining stage. Specifically, I went looking for the magic bullet—the guarantees of recovery and the assurances. But I found none. Learn to recognize, for example, when you are bargaining. For example, "If this problem goes away, I'll <fill in the blank>." Use this knowledge to chart your progress. Eventually I touched on all of the stages. I suggest that you learn these stages and perhaps even research them a little.

The depression stage is inevitable. However, you should strive to move through the depression stage as quickly as is possible. It won't help anything, and frankly, no matter how you cut it, depression is a selfish thing that works to exclude everything and everyone but yourself. Depression is all about you, and only you, not your child. The allergy is not about you, so getting depressed will only result in a failure to act positively and decisively, which is your job as a parent. If serious depression is triggered by your child's allergies and you cannot get past it, I would surmise that there is some other underlying problem for which you should seek help. Your child will need everything you can give them. You cannot help them if you are depressed.

I admit that I felt depressed. But I recognized it relatively quickly based upon my family history. Recognizing the depression told me where I was in the overall process and was actually cause for hope since I knew the next stages would be positive ones. This is where understanding the grief cycle and process of coping can be very helpful. It can act as a feedback mechanism that allows you to gauge where you are in the overall process and to use that knowledge to advance towards the next stage.

I passed through the depression stage relatively quickly and progressed into testing stage. During this stage, I learned the most and came to understand food allergies and their severity. I want to stress that I am still learning about the situation daily. As my children grow and mature, I know there will be new issues and challenges with respect to their food allergies. Because I realize this, I don't claim to understand all of the ramifications fully. The situation is fluid and changing. If I said I fully understand food allergies, then I would be incapable of learning and growing.

This process helped me reach the acceptance stage. I would say that perhaps the most important part of reaching acceptance is coming to understand as much as you can about food allergies, and in particular your children's allergies. It is difficult and painful, but it will help you to reach acceptance. Strive to reach acceptance. In this phase, you can make good decisions about the health of your children and yourself. I can say truly that once I reached acceptance and a fundamental understanding of food allergies, I began to feel relieved and a big burden was lifted.

One of the things about the phases of grief is that while you tend to be predominantly in one phase at a given time, you tend to circle back and forward at times, revisiting the earlier phases and reaching out into the next. It is important to remember that others will also go though these stages and that everyone will tend to react to them differently and progress at different rates. Be a leader. Try to understand the stages and learn to recognize where your loved ones are in this process and help them through it.

This process enhances the healing. For instance, once I began to understand the food allergies more fully, I could rationally think through what needed to be done. I was not as stressed anymore. Further I was capable of acting appropriately and decisively to mitigate risk and provide a safe environment for my children. Do I stress sometime still? Yes. Don't all parents? Does the subject of my children's food allergies fill me with dread and an all consuming fear? Do I lose sleep at night over it? Not any longer. I know my role and am prepared and competent.

When my second son was born, he had food allergies as well. We could not test immediately, and we hoped that perhaps he would not have food allergies. Later testing revealed that he had the same allergies as my first son. By the time we were certain of this however, we were well versed in the routine of establishing and keeping an allergen-free zone at home and mitigating risk outside the home. Little changed other than that we needed to watch two boys closely, especially when outside the home.

One important footnote to this however, is that you should not fully trust anyone, including health care providers, to do the right things or to understand the implications of food allergies and act accordingly. When my wife and I went to the hospital to give birth to our second son, the nurses were told that my wife would breastfeed the child. Moreover, I am certain that my wife's chart must have shown that we had a child with food allergies. The doctors that attended my wife certainly knew. Despite these things the nurses gave our second son *milk-based* formula the day he was born. I personally think it was sloppiness on everyone's part, and I should have been much more proactive. Be explicit with everyone about food allergies in the family. Get explicit acknowledgement of the seriousness of the situation and if the child will be outside of your control at any time, ask for details as to how everyone who could handle your children will be made aware of the condition.

The entire food allergy experience has been overall a positive one in some very real respects. Fatherhood generally has affected me positively and the food allergy factor has not detracted from this benefit. As a parent, and particularly as a father, my job is to mitigate risk, and to see to it that my children live long, healthy lives. Nothing brought out the truth of my job as a father as much as the food allergies. It made life very, very clear to me. It has lent a clarity and purpose to my life that I perhaps only faintly experienced prior to having children. In short, the entire experience has made me a more whole person.

There are a large number of changes that I have had to make which have been most gratifying and are worth mentioning. Since our children are allergic to dairy and eggs (no longer chicken) we've had to modify our own diets. In the beginning, we tried segregating foods. For example, we still had butter around but tried to keep it away from our children. But it became difficult to guarantee that we would not cross contaminate things. The stress generated from trying was way too much to handle. For example, my wife accidentally cut a grape up once where the knife had previously been used in butter, and our son developed hives from the invisible butter left on the knife. Additionally, we learned that cooking eggs sent the allergens into the air. Once we knew that, we decided to make our home an allergen-free zone. This was the best remedy to lower our stress levels.

To accomplish an allergen-free home, we learned all of the various aliases and names of ingredients that contain or are made from dairy and eggs. We started reading labels from top to bottom. Gradually, something amazing started to happen. We got sick of reading long lists of ingredients. Bit by bit, the ingredients lists got shorter and shorter until almost everything we purchased had only three or four ingredients. Further, we avoided foods that might be subject to cross contamination at the factory, by noting the allergen warnings on the label. With shorter ingredient lists, came healthier foods. As a natural part of this, we now eat mostly preservative-free foods. Gradually, that gave way to eating as many organic products as possible. Finally, better overall health has come with this healthier diet—I've lost fifty pounds since my first son was born. Yes, *fifty* pounds. I started to exercise, but I am confident that at least ten pounds, if not more, was lost due to not eating dairy. Also, I experienced something of a feedback cycle wherein as I started eating healthier, I wanted to be healthier. Another positive was that my improved health may have improved my work habits and possibly my career.

While my children's food allergies may have actually improved my health, there was and remains a hurdle to get over with family and friends when dealing with food. The truth is that few people understand it, and most people think that we are overreacting. So it takes some time. Eventually, most come to understand. Patience, persistence, and education are the key.

My biggest concern at present is the social ramifications of food allergies for our children. It is hard to both keep them active socially and to mitigate risk. When we go to birthday parties, we try not to make a big deal about not eating what everyone else is eating. Early on we substituted cake without telling our sons. Lately our eldest has started to ask his mother for "his" cake. He has been briefed on his allergies and can recite which allergies he has. Moreover, he seems truly to understand that he cannot eat certain foods and that Mom's cake is safe.

Perhaps our worst nightmare is the "pizza party." Greasy cheese gets all over everything and hot cheese tends to be airborne in trace amounts, and it is simply impossible to substitute. While we do avoid pizza parties, going overboard with our rules will inevitably result in fewer activities for our boys. As with anything in life, the key seems to be balance. Add to that some well informed vigilance, and food allergies need not necessarily curtail meaningful and fun contact with peers.

How is this all going to play out later in life when they enter school? I don't have the answers—yet. But I do know that if you control your stress levels, remain vigilant, and use the opportunity educate your children, for the most part it should be fine. If you are really worried about exposure from trace food contamination, and your child is not taking regular medication, then ask your doctor/allergist if you might perhaps give your child a little antihistamine in advance of any risky situation.

Another way to mitigate stress and worry is to join or start a group for parents of allergic children. Really get to know these other parents. You'll have much in common with them, and if there are social events, it will be safer and just as much fun. The kids, too, will come to understand that they are not all that different because there are others with food allergies. Perhaps, when the time comes at school, they will help each other.

Helping each other is the best way my wife and I support each other. I try to be as informed as I possibly can about food allergies and ingredients. I take the allergies seriously and try to provide my wife with a backup at every point. I feel strongly that the best way to help my wife is to get with the program, and more than that, to improve the program. Simply being on the team means there is a team. This will lighten her load significantly. Again, as the husband, one of my jobs is risk mitigation. We both cross-check each other constantly on ingredient lists, and render appropriate reminders to make sure we bring the EpiPen® Jr. on outings.

More than that though, I view my role as one of moral support. Trust me—your wife needs to have her load lightened. Remember that as you go through the stages described above, she will, too. There was a period during which my wife was in despair. She had hit the depression phase. I was closer to acceptance at that time and was able to lend some valuable perspective. It is important to try to bring the other person along wherever you can. In trying to bring the other person to a positive place, often you bring yourself to a more positive place. I have reminded her many times that everyone gets a bag of hammers in life to drag around. Our bag of hammers is serious and weighty but others have a harder time, a bigger bag of hammers. It helps to see that we have blessings too. In reminding her, I am also reminded. It always makes me feel better.

The hardest part overall was simply getting to acceptance. I cycled through the stages several times. Now it's just a way of life. I like our life. The second hardest part was getting past the initial stress that I felt. It was sort of a stifling fear and overbearing dread of something going wrong. The biggest help with that fear was to remove the allergens from our home. Perhaps the hardest lingering feeling is the doubt about their going to school and the social impact they may encounter at some point. But that is beyond our immediate control. We will cross those bridges when we get to them. I am sure that the experiences I am having now, each day, will inform our decisions then, and that they will be good ones.

If you find yourself in a similar situation, my advice to you is:

- *Take the food allergies seriously.* They are serious business. The sooner you accept that and your proper role as a father, the better your children will fare.

- *Learn everything you can about food allergies.* You need to understand food allergies to do your job as a father well.

- *Food allergies are not a weakness or a defect.* They are more common than you might think.

- *Your children's food allergies are not about you.* Get to a place where you can and do act positively and decisively for the good of your children. Whatever happens, get to testing/acceptance as fast as you can. You are of no use to your children or yourself bemoaning the cold, hard facts. Find something positive in the situation.

- *Back your wife up 110% (not just 100%).* Help her get through it too. She'll have a hard time, especially in the beginning. Don't make it harder. You need to present a unified face to the world in order to effectively deal with the issues that will arise.

- *Reduce risk by being a leader.* Don't stress-out, just make sure that the chances for exposure are minimal.

- *Find something or many things positive in the situation.* Be something positive in the situation.

The realization of the fact that our children have food allergies has been positive in many ways. Our diet has changed much for the better. I have learned to manage stress a little better. I've become more sure and steady as a father and know my job as a father better. I've grown a lot as a result of this. Before I had children I was self-absorbed. I have come to trust my wife more. I see just how hard she works at all of this and I am in awe. I like who I have become and who I am becoming as a father, and the allergies have been a part of the experience every step of the way. If this is our bag of hammers, I'll take it. I've seen the bag of hammers others have been given—it could be much worse. Food allergies are hardly a blessing. However, the changes that we have made to accommodate the food allergies have all been positive in some respect. In the final analysis, our children are thriving. They are happy and healthy. We are truly twice blessed.

Diet

INTRODUCTION

Avoiding allergens can be difficult. As mentioned, often it requires re-thinking how you grocery shop and cook. The easiest way to avoid allergens is to stick to the basics: fresh fruits, fresh vegetables, plain meat, unprocessed rice and potatoes.

Appetizers can include fresh fruit, vegetables, olives and unflavored corn or potato chips. Check the ingredients carefully and only buy ones with known ingredients that don't include unknowns such as natural flavors or artificial colors. Look closely for warnings and allergen notices.

Breakfast foods can include fresh fruits, whole grain breads and breakfast meats, such as bacon or ham. When preparing fresh fruit and vegetables wash them well by spraying and rubbing lemon juice to cut the pesticides or bacteria on the skins and be sure to rinse it well. Many cereals contain dairy and trace amounts of peanuts or tree nuts. Even trace amounts should be avoided. Cereals are also usually high in sugar. When I give my children a breakfast of bacon, whole grain bagels and some apple, they seem happier for a longer time as compared to a breakfast of cereal.

Lunch foods can include sandwiches with fresh fruits or vegetables and a snack food. I give my children potato chips or pretzels too. Even though these can be high in fat, the ingredients only include potatoes, oil and salt, so there are not a lot of preservatives.

For dinner, I prepare a meal of meat, vegetable and starch using natural, unprepared foods. For instance, I might make chicken sautéed in soy sauce with broccoli and brown rice or meatloaf (without egg) with mashed or roasted potatoes and corn.

Desserts can be the most difficult. Consider a fresh fruit salad for dessert or a plain homemade cake such as the one referenced in the "Birthday Party" section of this book. I have found that I need to bake desserts from scratch to be sure they are allergen-free. There are a lot of recipes on the Internet. Normally you can use an egg substitute or leave the egg out completely if only one egg is called for.

If you need to cook for someone with a food allergy, don't be shy about asking for a list of what they can or can't eat. Then consider the following when you grocery shop with your allergen list in hand:

- Don't buy prepackaged meats, starches or vegetables, like scalloped potatoes, rice pilaf, chicken cordon blue, or seasoned frozen vegetables like green beans with sliced almonds.

- Don't buy cookies, crackers, cakes and breads that contain lengthy ingredient lists because you might encounter allergens under hidden names, such as lactic acid (dairy) or arachis oil (peanut oil).

- Don't buy your meat in the deli if your children have dairy allergies. There is simply too much chance for cross contamination with cheese and other dairy products. Instead, purchase small hams and meat slabs that can be made into sandwiches by slicing at home.

- Do spend a lot of time in the fruit and vegetable aisle. Steaming fresh vegetables usually works well for people with allergies.

- Do purchase meats that are not prepared or seasoned. When cooking the meat try using only simple ingredients like oil, salt and pepper and try grilling or baking.

- Do try plain rice and potatoes. Buy a bag of plain brown rice and a bag of uncooked potatoes in the vegetable aisle. Don't add any seasoning to the rice except for salt. Potatoes can be baked or roasted with oil and salt.

CHAPTER 38: IDENTIFY THE BIG EIGHT ALLERGENS

Ninety percent of food allergies are caused by eight foods: Dairy, soy, egg, wheat, peanuts, tree nuts, fish and shellfish.[97] To help Americans avoid foods to which they are allergic, the Food Allergen Labeling and Consumer Protection Act of 2004 (FALCPA) was signed into law on August 2, 2004. According to the Food Allergy Initiative, "The Food Allergy Initiative celebrated a major victory in its public policy campaign when President George W. Bush signed the Food Allergen Labeling and Consumer Protection Act (S. 741) into law...The new law, effective January 1, 2006, will provide necessary information for school nurses, teachers, caregivers and chefs who must help millions of food allergic students and restaurant patrons avoid the food allergens...The bill requires food manufacturers to clearly state if a product contains any of the eight major food allergens responsible for over ninety percent of all allergic reactions; those allergens are dairy, eggs, peanuts, tree nuts, fish, shellfish, wheat, and soy. In addition, it requires that the Food and Drug Administration conduct inspections and issue a report within eighteen months to ensure that the food manufacturers comply with practices to reduce or eliminate cross-contact of a food with any major food allergens that are not intentional ingredients of the food."[98]

But beware of a few things: Products that were packaged prior to January 1, 2006, that may still be "on the shelf" will not carry the allergen label. Be alert to products that are packaged out of the country because they may not adhere to these labeling laws and, therefore, may contain hidden allergens. A prudent parent should always scan the ingredients list for allergens and other ingredient names that contain the allergens.

In regard to this third warning, I have compiled the following lists of ingredients which contain the allergens. These lists are not necessarily exhaustive but can serve as a starting point for you to create your own list by checking with your doctors and doing additional research to ensure that nothing on your child's plate or in your house, will contain allergy causing ingredients. Keep a list of ingredients to avoid in your wallet.

Dairy

Dairy includes all milk, cheese and by-products from cow's milk. Dairy is often divided into two types: lactose (the sugar) and casein (the protein). Lactose intolerance is not an allergy and while it can be uncomfortable for the digestive system, it will not produce anaphylactic shock.[99] Lactose-free (dairy-sugar-free) dairy products still contain dairy protein so lactose-free foods should *not* be consumed by those allergic to dairy.

To make matters more complicated, some products are labeled as "non-dairy" but contain dairy in the form of casein. Casein is cow's milk protein which is exactly what a child reacts to when an anaphylactic response is triggered. So a parent might pick up some rice cheese that says "non-dairy" on the front label, but the ingredient label might include casein, which is dairy protein. Therefore this "non-dairy" rice cheese could cause anaphylactic shock if fed to a child who is allergic to dairy. I have learned this from experience. Although I have never accidentally fed my children this kind of "non-dairy" cheese, there have been plenty of times I have stood in the grocery store reading the back label of a "non-dairy" cheese and found the milk protein or casein ingredient. I think it is wrong that manufacturers can market their products this way because it is misleading and dangerous. I saw a news story on television where a mother accidentally gave her pre-teen son this kind of cheese and it produced an allergic reaction.

I have found through my own experience of reading labels that dairy is included in almost all pre-packaged cakes, cookies, crackers, breads and cereals. It is commonly under the name of non-fat milk, lactic acid or whey in these products. I have found that any product which says, "calcium enriched" normally uses dairy as the source of that supplement. For instance calcium lactate can be found in apple juice and orange juice that says calcium enriched.

My husband discovered that some deli meats and hot dogs contain dairy from the processing stage. Even some tuna fish contains dairy. He asked our local supermarket deli service people whether the meat-slicers are used to slice both meat and cheese. They responded that they try to use one for meat and one for cheese, but if the cheese slicer is busy, they will slice the cheese on the slicer normally used for meat. So we don't buy meat from the deli for our sons because it may contain cheese residue.

I have found that some cosmetics, hair products, soaps, and lotions contain dairy products. For instance, I was using hair products and found that they contained lactic acid, a dairy ingredient. I stopped using these products because perhaps some dairy residue was being left around the house from my hair.

Dairy is or maybe in all of these ingredient names as well: Artificial flavoring (maybe), beverage whitener, butter, butter oil, calcium caseinate, calcium lactate, caramel, casein, caseinate, cheese, cream, custard, curd, demineralised whey, fromage frais, galactose, ghee, lactobacillus (unless specified that derived from a non-dairy source), lactalbumin phosphate, lactalbumin, lactate, lactic acid, lactoglobulin, milk powder, lactose, malted milk, margarine, milk solids, natural flavoring/flavors (maybe), non-fat milk, non-fat milk solids, potassium caseinate, ready sponge, skim milk powder, sodium caseinate, sour cream, sweet whey powder, vegetable fats, whey, whey protein, whey solids, yogurt.

There may be other ingredients that contain dairy or are derived from dairy. Please use this list as a starting point only, not as a comprehensive list. The information is general in nature and is provided for informational purposes only. Be sure to verify your list with your child's doctor. The above ingredient lists were obtained from various sources.[100] [101] [102]

Egg

Egg is not dairy even though you often find eggs in the dairy section in the grocery store. Dairy comes from cows. Eggs come from chickens. Egg substitutes often contain egg whites. Many pastas contain egg. Some specialty drinks contain eggs such as eggnog, apricot lady, mocha flip, tequila cocktail and hundreds of other mixed drinks.

Egg is or may be in all of these ingredient names: Albumin, egg solids, egg white, egg white solids, egg yolk, globulin, lecithin (maybe), livetin, lysozyme, ovalbumin, ovoglobulin, ovomucin, ovomucoid, ovotransferrin, ovovitelia, ovovitellin, powdered egg, silici albuminate, simplesse, vitellin, whole egg.

There may be other ingredients that contain egg or are derived from egg. Please use this list as a starting point only, not as a comprehensive list. The information is general in nature and is provided for informational purposes only. Be sure to verify your list with your child's doctor. The above ingredient lists were obtained from various sources.[103] [104]

Peanut

People who have a peanut allergy need to be vigilant to avoid peanuts and trace amounts of peanuts that might contaminate otherwise safe food. Trace contamination might occur when the same equipment is used to create a peanut food and a non-peanut food. Foods likely to be contaminated through manufacturing include: Chocolate candies, foreign restaurant foods (African, Chinese, Indonesian, Mexican, Thai and Vietnamese), bakery goods, ice cream, sunflower seeds, nut butters, health food bars, bouillon, Worcestershire sauce, praline, nougat, muesli, and chili.

Furthermore, non-food items might contain peanuts and should be avoided. These might include: Hackysacks, beanbags, draft dodgers, bird feed, dog food and treats, hamster food and bedding, livestock feed, secondhand toys and furniture, ant traps, mouse traps, and some cosmetics.

A 2006 article entitled, *Clarins Comes Under Fire over Peanut Ingredient* states, "Most people are aware that a variety of processed foods include peanuts or peanut-based ingredients, but far fewer are aware that cosmetic products also contain such ingredients. Hydrogenated peanut oil is, according to the NTEF, a key ingredient in sunscreen products, and specifically features in Clarins' Protection Sun Control Stick."[105]

Peanut is or may be in all of these ingredient names: Arachis, arachis oil (peanut oil), artificial flavoring (maybe), artificial nuts, emulsified [foods], food additive 322, Goobers, hydrolyzed vegetable protein, lecithin, mandelonas, marzipan, mixed nuts, monkey nuts, natural flavoring (maybe), nutmeat, peanut butter, pesto, and satay.

There may be other ingredients that contain peanuts or are derived from peanuts. Please use this list as a starting point only, not as a comprehensive list. The information is general in nature and is provided for informational purposes only. Be sure to verify your list with your child's doctor. The above ingredient lists were obtained from various sources.[106] [107] [108]

Tree Nut

People who have a tree nut allergy need to be vigilant to avoid tree nuts and any trace amounts of tree nuts that might contaminate otherwise safe food. Trace contamination might occur when the same equipment is used to create a tree nut food and a non-tree nut food. The tree nuts include: Almonds, Brazil nuts, cashews, hazelnuts (filberts), macadamia nuts, pecans, pine nuts (pignolias), pistachio nuts and walnuts. Peanuts are part of the legume family and are not considered a tree nut.

Foods likely to be contaminated through manufacturing include: Chocolate candies, foreign restaurant foods (African, Chinese, Indonesian, Mexican, Thai and Vietnamese), bakery goods, ice cream, sunflower seeds, nut butters, health food bars, bouillon, Worcestershire sauce, muesli, bakery goods, salad dressings, gravies, and trail mixes.

Furthermore, non-food items might contain tree nuts and should be avoided. These might include: Hackysacks, beanbags, draft dodgers, bird feed, dog food and treats, hamster food and bedding, livestock feed, hair products, sun screens, and massage oils.

Tree nuts are or may be in all of these ingredient names: Amaretto, anacardium nuts, artificial flavorings (maybe), artificial nuts, calisson, cashew butter, Frangelico®, gianduja, hickory nuts, marzipan, mortadella, natural flavorings (maybe), nougat, nut flavored coffee (like hazelnut coffee), nut butters, nut paste, nut meat, pesto, pinon, praline, queensland nut, as well as the basic nut names: Almonds, Brazil nuts, cashews, hazelnuts (filberts), macadamia nuts, pecans (mashugas), pine nuts (pignolias or pinyons), pistachio nuts and walnuts.

There may be other ingredients that contain tree nuts or are derived from tree nuts. Please use this list as a starting point only, not as a comprehensive list. The information is general in nature and is provided for informational purposes only. Be sure to verify your list with your child's doctor. The above ingredient lists were obtained from various sources.[109] [110] [111]

Soy

"Almost sixty percent of processed foods have soy in their ingredient list. Many people allergic to soy (a legume) are also allergic to other legumes such as peas, peanuts, lentils and garbanzo beans. Research has been done on soy allergies. Using a 'gene silencing' technique, researchers were able to 'knock out' a gene that makes a protein called P34, which is thought to trigger most allergic reactions to soy. Eliot Herman, Ph.D., U.S. Department of Agriculture's Agricultural Research Service states, 'There are up to fifteen different proteins in soybeans that people are allergic to...[t]he major one, P34, is responsible for seventy-five percent of the allergic reactions.'"[112]

Soy can be found in foods such as chicken broth, vegetable broth, gum, and starch, bouillon cubes (beef, chicken, vegetable, etc.), canned tuna, cereals, crackers, infant formulas, sauces, soups and can be found in peanut butter and other foods under the name of hydrolyzed vegetable protein (HVP), as well as natural flavoring and artificial flavoring.

Soy is or may be in all of these ingredient names: Artificial flavoring (maybe), edamame, lecithin, miso, natto, natural flavoring (maybe), shoyu sauce, soy, soy albumin, soy fiber, soy flour, soy grits, soy milk, soy nuts, soy sprouts, soya, soybean, soybean curd, soybean granules, soybean butter, soy protein, soy protein isolate, soy sauce, tamari, tempeh, textured vegetable protein (TVP) and tofu.

There may be other ingredients that contain soy or are derived from soy. Please use this list as a starting point only, not as a comprehensive list. The information is general in nature and is provided for informational purposes only. Be sure to verify your list with your child's doctor. The above ingredient lists were obtained from various sources.[113] [114]

Wheat

People who should avoid wheat include both those with celiac disease and an allergy to wheat. According to FAAN's Tips for managing a wheat allergy, Celiac disease and wheat allergy are two distinct conditions:

- *Wheat Allergy* is an allergy to wheat where an IgE-mediated response to wheat protein exists. These individuals must only avoid wheat. Most wheat-allergic children outgrow the allergy.[115]
- *Celiac Disease* is intolerance to gluten. The major grains that contain gluten are wheat, rye, oats and barley. These grains and their by-products must be strictly avoided by people with celiac disease. Celiac disease is a permanent (lifelong) adverse reaction to gluten.[116]

Wheat can be found in most pre-packaged cakes, cookies, candies, crackers, cereals, breads, waffles, pancakes, dumplings, muffins, cornbread, potato bread, soybean bread as well as grains, pastas, cereals and many processed foods that contain modified food starch, preservatives, and stabilizers such as gravy, pudding, cottage cheese or salad dressing. Sometimes it is found in medications as gluten. Wheat can be used in Asian dishes as a meat substitute and in some hot dogs, bologna, sausage, imitation crab meat and some ice creams. Some beverages can include wheat including cereal beverages, coffee substitutes, and instant chocolate drink mixes.

Wheat ingredients include: Ale, beer, bran, bread crumbs, cereal extract, couscous, cracked wheat, cracker meal, einkorn, emmer, enriched flour, farina, flour, gelatinized starch (maybe), gluten, graham, graham flour, gum (maybe), high gluten flour, high protein flour, hydrolyzed vegetable protein (maybe), hydrolyzed wheat protein, kamut, malt, modified food starch (maybe), monosodium glutamate (MSG), natural flavoring (maybe), root beer, semolina, soy sauce (maybe), spelt, triticale (a cross between wheat and rye), vegetable starch (maybe), vital gluten, wheat bran, wheat germ, wheat gluten, wheat malt, wheat starch, whole wheat flour and Worcestershire sauce.

Celiac Disease is an intolerance to gluten (wheat, rye, oat and barley). Celiac disease can appear with a variety of symptoms, with irritability as one of the most common symptoms in children, which makes it difficult to diagnose in children under five years. "People who have celiac disease cannot tolerate a protein called gluten, found in wheat, rye, oat and barley. When people with celiac disease eat foods or use products containing gluten, their immune system responds by damaging the small intestine. The tiny, fingerlike protrusions lining the small intestine (villi) are damaged or destroyed, which normally allow nutrients from food to be absorbed into the bloodstream. Without healthy villi, a person becomes malnourished, regardless of the quantity of food eaten," according to National Digestive Disease Clearinghouse.[117]

Complications from celiac disease include, "Damage to the small intestine and the resulting nutrient absorption problems [that] put a person with celiac disease at risk for malnutrition, anemia, and several other diseases and health problems. [These problems include] Lymphoma and adenocarcinoma—cancers that can develop in the intestine. Osteoporosis is a condition in which the bones become weak, brittle, and prone to breaking. Poor calcium absorption contributes to osteoporosis. Miscarriage and congenital malformation of the baby, such as neural tube defects, are risks for pregnant women with untreated celiac disease because of nutrient absorption problems. Short stature refers to being significantly under the average height. Short stature results when childhood celiac disease prevents nutrient absorption during the years when nutrition is critical to a child's normal growth and development. Children who are diagnosed and treated before their growth stops may have a catch-up period."[118]

If you are avoiding gluten altogether, the following list of wheat, rye, oat and barley foods can be used as a starting point: Abyssinian hard (wheat triticum duran), avena (wild oat), barley (hordeum vulgare), barley malt, barley extract, beer (ale, porter, stout, fermented beverages), blue cheese, bran, bread flour, broth, bulgur (bulgur wheat, bulgur nuts), bouillon, cereal (cereal extract, cereal binding), cracker meal, croutons, couscous, dinkle, durum, einkorn (wild einkorn), emmer (wild emmer), edible starch, farina, farro, filler, fu, flour (all-purpose, barley, bleached, bread, brown, durum, enriched, gluten, graham, granary, high protein, high gluten, oat, wheat, white), germ, gluten, glutenin, graham flour, hordeum, horderum vulgare, hydrolyzed oat starch, hydrolyzed wheat gluten, hydrolyzed wheat protein, kamut, malt, malt beverages, malt extract, malted milk, malt flavoring, malt syrup, malt vinegar, matzo (matzah), mir (wheat, rye), miso (may contain barley), mustard powder, oats, oat bran, oat fiber, oat gum, oat syrup, oriental wheat, rice malt, rice syrup, brown rice syrup, rye, scotch, soy sauce, seitan, semolina, spelt, sprouted wheat, tabbuleah, triticale, udon, vital gluten, wheat, wheat berry, wheat bran, wheat germ, wheat germ oil, wheat grass, wheat gluten, wheat starch, and whole wheat berries.[119]

There may be other ingredients that contain wheat, rye, oat, barley or gluten. Please use this list as a starting point only, not as a comprehensive list. The information is general in nature and is provided for informational purposes only. Be sure to verify your list with your child's doctor. The above ingredient lists were obtained from various sources.[120]

Fish and Shellfish

According to the Food Allergy and Anaphylaxis Network, "Allergic reactions to fish and shellfish can be severe and are often a cause of anaphylaxis. Fish-allergic individuals should avoid fish and seafood restaurants because of the risk of contamination in the food preparation area of their "non-fish" meal from a counter, spatula, cooking oil, fryer, or grill exposed to fish. Fish protein can become airborne during cooking and cause an allergic reaction. Some individuals have had reactions from walking through a fish market."[121] Unfortunately, seafood allergies are life-long.[122]

Several years ago, I remember being surprised when I read the ingredient label of a frozen *turkey* dinner with vegetables and noticed there was *fish* in the sauce, "How strange," I thought. Strange or not, fish and shellfish can be found in many items that you might not expect, including: Gelatin, salad dressings, meat sauces, marinara sauce, hot dogs, deli meats, chili, vitamins, and frozen dinners. Fish and shellfish are common in many types of foods, especially Asian food, Thai food, Chinese food, Japanese food and Vietnamese food.

Fish and shellfish ingredients include: Agar, alfonsinos or golden eye perch, alginate, alginic acid, american plaice, anchovies, anglerfish, black scabbardfish, blue ling, bouillabaisse, brill, caviar, chilean seabass, clams, cockle, cod, crab, crawfish, crayfish, daikon cake, disodium ionsinate, dogfish, eel, fish, fish balls, fish oils, fish sauce, fish soup, fish/shellfish flavoring, frito misto, fruits de mer, glucosamine hcl, greater forkbeard, grouper, gumbo, haddock, hake, halibut, haw gow, herring, imitation crabmeat, langoustine, ling, lobster, marlin, monkfish, mussels, nursehound, ocean perch, omega-3 supplements, orange roughy, oysters, paella, patagonian toothfish, plaice, prawn, rat fish, rabbit fish, ray fish, redfish, roe, roundnose grenadier, salmon, sashimi, scallops, sea urchin, seabass, seabream, shark, shrimp, shrimp balls, silver smelt, skate, snapper, spurdog, sturgeon, sui my, surimi, sushi, swordfish, taro cake, tempura, tiger prawn, torsk, tuna, turbot, tusk, wolffish, and Worcestershire sauce.

If you are allergic to a kind of fish or shellfish, you may or may not be allergic to other kinds of fish or shellfish. There are "around 13,000 common names...for the 4,482 named species of fishes currently known from Australian waters," according to the Australian Museum Fish site.[123]

There may be other ingredients that contain fish and shellfish. Please use this list as a starting point only, not as a comprehensive list. The information is general in nature and is provided for informational purposes only. Be sure to verify your list with your child's doctor. The above ingredient lists were obtained from various sources.[124] [125] [126]

CHAPTER 39: ARTIFICIAL OR NATURAL INGREDIENTS

In addition to avoiding the allergen(s), described in the previous chapter, to which your child is allergic, I recommend avoiding natural flavors, natural colors, artificial flavors and artificial colors. The new labeling laws state that allergens should be listed in bold print if included in these catch-all ingredient names, but I question whether the law is being adhered to and why such a catch-all ingredient is even in a food product. Why not list all the ingredients separately? What is there to hide? Further, who is doing quality assurance on these products to ensure allergens are not included in these catch-all ingredients? I researched the exact definitions of natural/artificial flavors, natural/artificial colors and spices in Title 21 of the Food and Drug Administration code.

Natural Flavors or Flavoring

"The term natural flavor or natural flavoring means the essential oil, oleoresin, essence or extractive, protein hydrolysate, distillate, or any product of roasting, heating or enzymolysis, which contains the flavoring constituents derived from a spice, fruit or fruit juice, vegetable or vegetable juice, edible yeast, herb, bark, bud, root, leaf or similar plant material, meat, seafood, poultry, eggs, dairy products, or fermentation products thereof, whose significant function in food is flavoring rather than nutritional."[127] Therefore, it appears that natural flavors can come from any source including the big eight allergens: Dairy, egg, soy, wheat, peanut, tree nut, fish and shellfish.

Artificial Flavors or Flavoring

"The term artificial flavor or artificial flavoring means any substance, the function of which is to impart flavor, which is not derived from a spice, fruit or fruit juice, vegetable or vegetable juice, edible yeast, herb, bark, bud, root, leaf or similar plant material, meat, fish, poultry, eggs, dairy products, or fermentation products thereof. Artificial flavor includes the substances listed in Secs. 172.515(b) and 182.60 of this chapter except where these are derived from natural sources."[128]

Since these laws allow for many chemicals and allergens to be placed in foods and not listed on the label specifically, we really don't know what we are eating and giving to our children. For example, according to *Fast Food Nation*, "A typical artificial strawberry flavor, like the kind found in a Burger King strawberry milk shake, contains the following ingredients: amyl acetate, amyl butyrate, amyl valerate, anethol, anisyl formate, benzyl acetate, benzyl isobutyrate, butyric acid, cinnamyl isobutyrate, cinnamyl valerate, cognac essential oil, diacetyl, dipropyl ketone, ethyl acetate, ethyl amyl ketone, ethyl butyrate, ethyl cinnamate, ethyl heptanoate, ethyl heptylate, ethyl lactate, ethyl methylphenylglycidate, ethyl nitrate, ethyl propionate, ethyl valerate, heliotropin, hydroxyphenyl-2-butanone (10 percent solution in alcohol), a-ionone, isobutyl anthranilate, isobutyl butyrate, lemon essential oil, maltol, 4-methylacetophenone, methyl anthranilate, methyl benzoate, methyl cinnamate, methyl heptine carbonate, methyl naphthyl ketone, methyl salicylate, mint essential oil, neroli essential oil, nerolin, neryl isobutyrate, orris butter, phenethyl alcohol, rose, rum ether, g-undecalactone, vanillin, and solvent."[129] There aren't even any strawberries in it.

Artificial and Natural Colors or Coloring

Have you ever noticed that organic fruits and vegetable appear less appetizing than the non-organic ones that have been sprayed with coloring? According to the U.S. Food and Drug Administration, color additives are used in foods, "to correct natural variations in color. Off-colored foods are often incorrectly associated with inferior quality. For example, some tree-ripened oranges are often sprayed with citrus red no.2 to correct the natural orangey-brown or mottled green color of their peels ([but] masking inferior quality, however, is an unacceptable use of colors)."[130] Whether the color has been used from a natural source (like one of the big eight allergens) or created in a test tube (perhaps like citrus red no. 2), I try to avoid them all.

"The term artificial color or artificial coloring means any 'color additive' as defined in Sec. 70.3(f) of this chapter," which is, "(f) A color additive is any material, not exempted under section 201(t) of the act, that is a dye, pigment, or other substance made by a process of synthesis or similar artifice, or extracted, isolated, or otherwise derived, with or without intermediate or final change of identity, *from a vegetable, animal, mineral, or other source* and that, when added or applied to a food, drug, or cosmetic or to the human body or any part thereof, is capable (alone or through reaction with another substance) of imparting a color thereto..."[131] Therefore, since artificial color can come from any source including vegetables and animals, it sounds like it includes the big eight allergens: Dairy, egg, soy, wheat, peanut, tree nut, fish and shellfish.

Even worse it states, "When a coloring has been added to butter, cheese, or ice cream, it need not be declared in the ingredient list unless such declaration is required by a regulation in part 73 or part 74 of this chapter to ensure safe conditions of use for the color additive. Voluntary declaration of all colorings added to butter, cheese, and ice cream, however, is recommended."[132] In other words, it appears the manufactures are not necessarily required to list *all* of the coloring added to foods.

Various reports describe the use of colorants in our foods, such as, "[B]eet juice, which provides a nice red color hue at slightly higher pH will undergo severe color loss when exposed to heat. Certain vegetable juice products, however, are extremely resilient and provide excellent color stability under both heating processes and freeze-thaw cycles. While natural colorants offer increasing benefits and become less restrictive than artificial colors, they are also becoming more cost effective. Natural colors are usually very concentrated, resulting in low dosage levels (0.1-0.5 %) with no effect on texture or flavor. If desired, the colors can even be unitized with the flavors or incorporated into the fruit preparations. Natural colorants in dairy products are also very stable to heat and light with excellent shelf life stability."[133] "Food ingredients such as cherries, green or red peppers, chocolate, and orange juice which contribute their own natural color when mixed with other foods are not regarded as color additives; but where a food substance such as beet juice is deliberately used as a color, as in pink lemonade, it is a color additive."[134] Again, why can't manufacturers list each ingredient separately rather than lumping them into a catch-all ingredient like natural or artificial colors, coloring, or colorant? If it has beet juice, then put it in the ingredient list.

Spices

"The term spice means any aromatic vegetable substance in the whole, broken, or ground form, except for those substances which have been traditionally regarded as foods, such as onions, garlic and celery; whose significant function in food is seasoning rather than nutritional; that is true to name; and from which no portion of any volatile oil or other flavoring principle has been removed. Spices include the spices listed in Sec. 182.10 and part 184 of this chapter, such as the following: Allspice, anise, basil, bay leaves, caraway seed, cardamon, celery seed, chervil, cinnamon, cloves, coriander, cumin seed, dill seed, fennel seed, fenugreek, ginger, horseradish, mace, marjoram, mustard flour, nutmeg, oregano, paprika, parsley, pepper, black; pepper, white; pepper, red; rosemary, saffron, sage, savory, star aniseed, tarragon, thyme, turmeric. Paprika, turmeric, and saffron or other spices, which are also colors, shall be declared as 'spice and coloring' unless declared by their common or usual name."[135] Based upon this definition, I will buy foods that list spices in the ingredient name—although I would prefer they list each spice separately and that the spices be organic.

The bottom line for our family is that if a food label includes natural flavors, natural colors, artificial flavors or artificial colors, we stay away from it. I do this because I would speculate that it would be easy for manufacturers to omit ingredient information from the allergen label and not get caught. They should list each and every ingredient.

CHAPTER 40: CROSS-REACTIONARY SUBSTANCES

In addition to avoiding the foods to which a child is allergic and catch-all ingredients like natural and artificial flavors or colors, I suggest considering avoiding foods that have a reputation for being cross-reactive with the allergens you are avoiding. In doing so, consider a food's similarities to other foods. For instance, tree nuts include almonds, Brazil nuts, cashews, hazelnuts (filberts), macadamia nuts, pecans, pine nuts (pignolias), pistachio nuts and walnuts. Sometimes when a person is allergic to one of these nuts, he'll be allergic to all or several other nuts in the tree nut group. Shellfish is another allergen that includes many varieties in the same food group. If a person is allergic to one type of shellfish—crab for instance—then there is a likelihood that the allergy might exist for lobster, clams, shrimp and other types of shellfish. Furthermore, a person with a peanut allergy might react to other legumes such as soy, peas, lentils and beans. These reactions to several or many foods in the *same* group are known as "cross-reactivity."

A bit more perplexing is cross-reactivity between foods in *different* groups. "Cross-reactivity can be a particularly vexing problem because it allows novel allergens, without warning, to elicit full-blown allergic symptoms...The problem frequently occurs among persons sensitive to peanuts...Though peanuts are *legumes*, they often foster a related sensitivity to *tree nuts*, such as almonds, filberts, and cashews."[136]

The following bulleted descriptions are examples of people who have had less common cross-reactions. They are reprinted here to help you maintain an inquisitive attitude if you encounter an odd reaction in you child. Consider exactly what your child ate or came into contact with, if an allergic-like response occurs. These examples are reprinted here with permission from Science News Online, copyright 1998:[137]

- A Houston-area man had been intrigued by the taste of mango smoothies, a pleasing drink he encountered on several recent visits to a friend's house. So when mangos went on sale at the local grocery store, this twenty-seven-year-old Texan decided to buy one. The tropical import has a thick green skin. To remove it, the man firmly grasped the fruit in his left hand, using his right to peel it. When the phone rang, the man sat down to answer it—without first washing his hands [and touched his thigh]. Three days later, an oozing, blistery rash broke out. While it resembled poison ivy—something he had experienced plenty of times during adolescence—the man could not fathom where he might have encountered the plant. So he showed the irritation to Mark O. Tucker and Chad R. Swan, residents in general surgery at St. Joseph Hospital, in Houston. They helped him to piece the puzzle together. Having been sensitized to poison ivy, the man's immune system was primed to respond to the plant's rash-inducing oleoresin. It apparently encountered that resin, or one nearly identical to it, in the mango's skin.

- A team of researchers from Bombay, India, published the first reports of persons with life-threatening allergies to fenugreek, a common spice derived from the seeds of a legume. Both affected women had a known allergy to chickpeas, another legume. Their coming from a related family of plants, the researchers said, suggests "[a] possible cross-reactivity between these two legumes."

- In another instance, a twenty-four-year-old Australian woman with an allergy to alcoholic beverages found herself hospitalized with wheezing, swelling of the lips and mouth, and a near loss of consciousness after eating rock melon. Despite having developed classic symptoms of anaphylactic shock, subsequent tests uncovered no evidence that the woman was actually allergic to the fruit. However, in probing further, her doctors learned that the particular melon that had evoked the life-threatening symptoms had tasted overripe and a bit pungent. They concluded that their patient's melon had begun to ferment—producing alcohol. In the March 1997 Annals of Allergy, Asthma, and Immunology, Dominic F.J. Mallon and Connie H. Katelaris, describe this as the first instance of alcohol-induced anaphylaxis stemming from overly ripe fruit.

- A thirty-six-year-old woman living in Madrid developed runny eyes and wheezing—evidence of allergic asthma—whenever she touched leaves of the weeping ficus (Ficus benjamina) plants in her home. Earlier this year, a team of immunologists reported that on three separate occasions, the woman's tongue and throat started to itch and swell up after eating: A fresh fig triggered one episode, a dried fig provoked a second; and kiwi fruit induced the third. María Luz Díez-Gómez and her colleagues at Madrid's Hospital Ramón y Cajal note that the fig plant (Ficus carica) is not closely related to the ornamental figs that flanked the woman's living room sofa for twelve years. However, the physicians did find evidence that the woman exhibited allergic responses to several enzymes present in the fruits—which may be a possible clue to their cross-reactivity with the ornamental ficus.

- Still other reports have highlighted instances in which persons with allergies to latex rubber subsequently developed a cross-reactivity to fruit (such as bananas) and individuals allergic to birch pollen exhibited an apparent cross-sensitivity to kiwi fruit.

Cross-reactions can be surprising and serious. Therefore, if your child already has one food allergy you should be on watch for additional food allergies. Introduce new foods with caution and be aware enough to recognize unusual reactions to new foods or items in the child's environment.

"In recent years, a number of immunologists have begun campaigning for thorough labeling of ingredients in commercially prepared foods.

The goal is to help persons with allergies identify products with the potential to trigger life-threatening reactions. However, these tougher labeling regulations would not shield people from exposures to all the host of compounds that may mimic their known allergens."[138] In other words, cross-reactive foods will not appear on food labels. If your child has food allergies, then research which foods might be similar by asking your child's doctor or doing research on the Internet or at the library.

Sometimes the link between cross-reactive foods is not clear. "A coconut is a seed of a fruit and nutmeg is obtained from the seeds of a tropical tree. Therefore, they are not usually restricted from the diet of someone allergic to tree nuts. However, some people have reacted to coconut and nutmeg. Consult your allergist before trying coconut or nutmeg products," if allergic to tree nuts.[139]

Other food reactions can be triggered by the presence of pollens in the air. For instance, if there is a lot of birch pollen or grass pollen in the air, then a food to which a person might not normally react, will in fact, cause a reaction. Birch pollen has similar protein qualities as those of some fruits and vegetables. It is not clear whether the traditional IgE antibody is created in these cases. The article states, "Moreover, IgE-binding proteins related to the birch pollen minor allergen Bet v 6 have been found in many vegetable foods such as apple, peach, orange, lychee fruit, strawberry, persimmon, zucchini, and carrot. Frequently, the occurrence of cross-reactive IgE antibodies is not correlated with the development of clinical food allergy."[140] It appears that people who have sensitive allergic reactions tend to react more to both environmental allergens and food allergens more often than those without any allergies.

"Another interesting example of cross-reactivity occurs in people who are highly sensitive to ragweed. During ragweed pollen season, they sometimes find that when they try to eat melons, particularly cantaloupe, they experience itching in their mouths and simply cannot eat the melon. Similarly, people who have severe birch pollen allergy also may react to apple peels. This is called the 'oral allergy syndrome.'"[141]

Sometimes people think that they have a cross-reactive allergy, but instead it is actually just a higher incidence of being allergic to similar things. For instance, "If one has a shellfish allergy, or any allergy for that matter, there is a slightly increased risk of iodine allergy. As compared to the person without an allergy to shellfish, people allergic to shellfish may show about a five percent greater chance of [exhibiting] iodine allergy symptoms. However similar studies show that having any [allergy] increases the chance of being sensitive to iodine."[142]

Nevertheless, although not a true cross-reaction, this likelihood should be kept in mind. I interviewed a woman named Ria, now 42, who survived a tough childhood in the 1960s due to severe food allergies and eczema. She was allergic to dairy, egg and lobster. She was also sensitive to over one hundred other allergens. She avoided cow's milk until she was seven and had her hands wrapped in gauze to keep from her habit of scratching the eczema at night until she bled. Doctors gave her cortisone shots every other week for four years and she recalls her aching arm and headaches.

Now Ria has allergies to lobster, artificial sweeteners and iodine. Once, Ria was to undergo some tests where doctors would inject some dye into her blood stream to see if she had any blockages or other abnormal structures in her internal organs. She lay in the bed with the needle in her arm and the doctor standing beside her. The doctor then said, "You did answer the questionnaire about allergies right?" Ria responded, "Yes, but no one asked me about iodine, which I am also allergic to." The doctor lunged for her arm and ripped the I.V. saying "This will kill you!" The dye solution was made of twenty-five percent iodine. She was fine, but it was a close call. Recently she decided to get a medical alert bracelet that will indicate her iodine allergy should she be unconscious and need medical attention.

Chapter 41: Allergy and Contact List

Once you identify you child's allergies and all of the hidden names and possible cross reactive foods or substances, I recommend making an emergency contact and allergy list.

I prepared the following document and emailed it to my neighbor, relatives, and close friends should there be an emergency and I am unable to care for our children. I also taped a copy of it to the inside of one of our cabinet doors where we keep a lot of snacks for our children. I always show it to the babysitters each time they come.

Parents:	Name	xxx-xxx-xxxx (phone)	
	Name	xxx-xxx-xxxx (phone)	
Friends:	Name	xxx-xxx-xxxx (phone)	
Family:	Name	xxx-xxx-xxxx (phone)	
Doctors:	Pediatrician:	xxx-xxx-xxxx	
	Allergist:	xxx-xxx-xxxx	
	Hospital:	xxx-xxx-xxxx	24-hour-number
	Local Police:	xxx-xxx-xxxx	

Allergies: Do not allow the boys to eat or handle any food, packaging or play item containing dairy, eggs, peanuts or any nut (see list on next page).

Reaction: Rash or hives on face around mouth and cough, like choking. A bad reaction prevents breathing, since the lips, tongue and throat will swell.

Response: _____ of antihistamine

- *or* -

EpiPen® Jr. in thigh muscle for 30 seconds (locations: master bathroom linen closet in blue medicine containers, or black bag in closet near laundry room).

	Egg Reaction Level (1-5)	Dairy Reaction Level (1-5)		Other Ingredients to Avoid
Name	3 (moderate)	3 (moderate)		
Name	5 (high)	3 (moderate)		
	Avoid egg ingredients including: albumin egg solids egg white egg white solids egg yolk globulin lecithin (maybe) livetin lysozyme ovalbumin ovoglobulin ovomucin ovomucoid ovotransferrin ovovitelia ovovitellin powdered egg silici albuminate simplesse vitellin whole egg	**Avoid dairy ingredients including:** beverage whitener butter butter oil calcium caseinate calcium lactate caramel casein caseinate cheese cream custard curd demineralised whey fromage frais galactose ghee lactobacillus lactalbumin phosphate lactalbumin lactate lactic acid lactoglobulin milk powder	lactose malted milk margarine milk solids non-fat milk non-fat milk solids potassium caseinate ready sponge skim milk powder sodium caseinate sour cream sweet whey powder vegetable fats whey whey protein whey solids yogurt Dairy probably does *not* include: calcium citrate calcium carbonate potassium lactate (maybe)	**Avoid all tree nuts and peanuts:** brazil nuts cashews hazelnuts (filberts) macadamia nuts peanuts pecans pine nuts (pignolias) pistachio nuts walnuts **Avoid:** natural flavors natural flavorings artificial flavors artificial flavorings natural colors natural colorings artificial colors artificial colorings

CHAPTER 42: PROBIOTICS ARE GOOD

One of the important secrets to enjoying young children is to have friends who have children who are generally the same age. Sharing frustrations, stories and laughter has helped me immensely as a new mother. In fact, just about one month before the birth of my second child, one of my friends and I planned a dinner out to celebrate. She too was pregnant and due at generally the same time. So we picked a date and a location and planned to have dinner out together.

We then invited a few other close friends to join us, and they agreed readily. Then we were at a BBQ with some additional friends when we were saying our good-byes when a few more friends wanted to join us as well. We welcomed them to the dinner. So we had the dinner and about ten or twelve moms showed up. It was great. We laughed and talked and ate. There were no interruptions. It was all about us. This was a nice change after focusing on others for a year or two. It felt like old times, pre-children, but with an additional connection—that of having children.

We had such a good time, we decided to try it again the next month. Then we tried it again the month after. Now almost three years later, we have barely missed one. We still meet the first Wednesday of every month and pick a new location for dinner. A different mom is in charge of picking the location and making the reservation each month. The dinners aren't just for fun...

It was at one of these dinners that a friend mentioned something for which I am extremely grateful. Our first son was about two and one-half years. We had learned about his allergies by this time. We also experienced several illnesses over the past year. When he was about six months old, he had strep throat, tracheal bronchitis and an ear infection. His doctor placed him on a nebulizer treatment and antibiotics. Over that year, he had several other illnesses, such as pneumonia, and required antibiotics a few times.

My friend pointed out that each time he was on antibiotics, the bacteria in his digestive system was destroyed. His little body had to rebuild the bacteria to be able to digest his food successfully. She suggested giving him some acidophilus, which was familiar to me in the form of yogurt. Since my son could not eat yogurt, because it is a dairy product, I began my search for dairy-free acidophilus.

That evening I did some research on acidophilus on the Internet. I learned something very interesting. Specifically, acidophilus might also help with my son's food allergies. I was thrilled. I felt that I had made an incredible discovery and had new hope for my son's ability to outgrow his food allergies and be healthier. The next day I called our allergist and asked her what she thought about the topic. She said that there have been some studies that have show that acidophilus might help the digestive system mature, thereby improving a child's ability to outgrow food allergies but it wasn't a cure. She said there were no real risks to giving him the acidophilus except to be sure that it was not derived from a dairy source.

I found some chewable tablets at the local health food store that were dairy-free acidophilus for children and began giving them to my son. I continued this from the fall when he was two and one-half years old to the spring when he was just over three. Then I did more research on the Internet and found some extremely interesting descriptions of the functions for each probiotic strain on Klaire Labs website.[143] (They do have a disclaimer stating that the following information has not been approved by the FDA. The following is reprinted with permission of Klaire Labs, a division of ProThera, Inc. Reno, NV.)

> *Lactobacillus acidophilus:* Highly resistant to gastric acid, bile, pepsin, and pancreatin. Possesses more than twenty known peptidases and breaks down casein and gluten. Ferments lactose and metabolizes a variety of other sugars and polysaccharides. Antagonizes a wide range of pathogenic bac-

teria. Reduces intestinal concentrations of carcinogenic enzymes.

Lactobacillus rhamnosus: Produces more peptidases than any other Lactobacillus species. Favorably enhances innate and acquired immunity. Inhibits proinflammatory cytokine production. Outstanding colon epithelial cell adherence. Suppresses pathogenic Escherichia coli internalization. Antagonizes rotavirus and Clostridium difficile. Supports gut microflora during antibiotic therapy. May support immune function in infants with allergies.

Lactobacillus casei: A hardy, adaptive transient species. Makes many proline-specific peptidases enhancing casein, casein-derived polypeptide, and gluten break down. Beneficially modulates innate immune responses. Increases the number of intestinal IgA-producing cells. Antagonizes Helicobacter pylori. Decreases proinflammatory cytokine secretion. Inhibits E. coli adherence to and invasion of intestinal cells. Decreases Shigella-mediated inflammation.

Lactobacillus salivarius: Indigenous to the intestinal tract and other mucosal surfaces. Secretes several anti-microbial agents. Reduces proinflammatory cytokine secretion. Attenuates inflammatory responses to Salmonella typhimurium. Stimulates interleukin-10 secretion, a cytokine inhibiting the inflammatory response to bacterial DNA. Enhances intestinal calcium uptake. Significantly supports intestinal barrier function.

Lactobacillus plantarum: A highly beneficial transient bacteria generally lacking in people consuming a standard Western diet while universally present in people consuming traditional plant-based diets. Exceedingly resistant to gastric acid and bile salts. Facilitates induction of the central regulatory cytokine, interleukin-12. Decreases production of inflammatory mediators. Supports intestinal barrier function. Reduces translocation of gut bacteria. Antagonizes C. difficile. Supports normal microflora in people with irritable bowel syndrome.

Lactobacillus paracasei: Excellent acid-tolerance. Highly resistant to pancreatin. Ferments inulin and phleins and produces high levels of lactic acid. Antagonizes C. difficile and Staphylococcus aureus as well as other pathogens. Contributes to a healthy vaginal microflora. Has supportive benefit in conditions ranging from allergic rhinitis to nonrotavirus diarrhea in children.

Lactobacillus brevis: A colonizing species producing lactate, carbon dioxide, ethanol, and acetate. Resistant to gastric acid, bile acids, and digestive enzymes. Excellent adherent properties. Increases production of interferon. Metabolically unique in the production of arginine deaminase to break down arginine and reduce polyamine production, compounds associated with vaginal dysbiosis and intestinal carcinogenesis.

Bifidobacterium bifidum: Present in large numbers in a healthy colon. Populations are reduced in allergic infants and decline significantly with age. Suppresses total and antigen-specific IgE production. Enhances IgM and IgG responses to select antigens. Activates B cell IgA secretion. Enhances IgA response to C. difficile toxin A. Along with L. acidophilus, supports gut microflora during antibiotic therapy and reduces positive testing for C. difficile toxins.

Bifidobacterium infantis: Frequently found in infants' intestinal tracts, but rarely in older adults. Strong suppressive effect on Bacteroides vulgatus, a commensal bacteria thought to have a role in inflammatory bowel disease. Reduces proinflammatory cytokine production. Supports normal microflora and inflammatory cytokine ratios in patients with irritable bowel syndrome. Together with L. acidophilus, supports the gut microflora in very low birth weight infants decreasing the risk of necrotizing enterocolitis and promotes normal microflora in children with diarrhea.

Bifidobacterium longum: Often the dominant Bifidobacterium species in humans. Ferments a broad spectrum of oligosaccharides. Resistant to high bile salt concentrations. Inhibits human neutrophil elastase which may be important to innate immunity and attenuate harmful intestinal inflammation. Inhibits enterotoxigenic E. coli receptor binding and translocation. Augments intestinal IgA secretory response to dietary proteins. Favorably modulates inflammatory cytokine response to respiratory antigens. Improves inflammation in ulcerative colitis.

Bifidobacterium breve: Secretes compounds, such as lactosidase, that favorably modify intestinal microflora by reducing Bacteroides and Clostridium concentrations and degrading mucin. Stimulates Peyer's patch B cell proliferation and antibody production. Eliminates stool Campylobacter jejuni in campylobacter enteritis restoring normal intestinal microflora. Antagonizes rotavirus and decreases rotavirus shedding in infants with rotavirus diarrhea.

Streptococcus thermophilus: A transient species with a long history of use as a starter culture for yogurt and cheese. Highly adapted to lactose metabolism. Many fermentation end-products including formate, acetoin, acetylaldehyde, diacetyl, and acetate that inhibit pathogenic bacterial proliferation. Reduces DNA damage and premalignant lesion formation by protecting against carcinogens. Along with other probiotics supports normal microflora and gastrointestinal function in conditions ranging from rotavirus diarrhea in infants to remission in ulcerative colitis.

Lactobacillus bulgaricus: A highly adapted, transient species closely related to *L.* acidophilus. Along with *S.* thermophilus, it has long been used in the production of yogurt and cheese. Supports normal cholesterol levels and reduces low density lipoprotein cholesterol oxidation. Suppresses proinflammatory cytokine production.

I decided to ask our allergist what she thought about each of these strains—would she recommend one or two, or perhaps advise me to stay away from some? She called me very soon after I sent the letter and said that she did not recommend a specific strain as a *cure* for the food allergies, since there is no scientific proof, but that I could give him a dose that contained the widest variety of strains. She also said that I could give him a full adult dose. She did not have any opinion about how (with food, water or juice) or when (morning, mid-day or evening) the dosage was administered. I began to give our son a full dose of the probiotics with the largest number of strains that were certified to be non-dairy.

Every morning I broke apart a full capsule and dumped the white powder contents into about one ounce of water which he drank before eating or drinking anything else in the morning. After about fifteen minutes, I would give him breakfast. My husband and I noticed some amazing results within about one week.

For the first time in his life, my son said he was hungry. Up until this point, it seemed as though he had trouble recognizing that he was hungry. He would then continue playing, without eating, until his low blood sugar would overcome him and he would become highly upset about something. These episodes were very frustrating to my husband and to me since we were not sure what would set him off. We loved our son so much and it caused a lot of pain to see him so unhappy at times. But now, because my son now seemed to miraculously recognize that he was hungry, he would eat. Since he would eat when he was hungry, his blood sugar level probably stabilized. I found his behavior improved significantly. He seemed happier, more stable and calmer. This was like a breath of fresh air for us.

In addition to the results of his learning to say that he was hungry and his improved behavior, we found he was not getting sick. He had a double ear infection and pneumonia right before starting this increased probiotics therapy (bigger dose with wider number of strains), but then he did not get sick again until the following winter, about nine months, when he got a mild to moderate sinus infection according to the doctor. We did put him on antibiotics again at that time but continued the probiotics regimen as well. In fact, our pediatrician advised us to increase the probiotics regimen by two or three times a day during the period of time that he was on the antibiotics and shortly thereafter. Now at age four and a few months our son has been healthy for the past year.

His growth improved as well. He had been average weight at birth, but had dropped to somewhere between tenth and thirtieth percentile for a few years. We were so worried about him when he was two—he was sick with pneumonia and so thin. Then, on the probiotics, he gained five pounds from age three to four and grew four and one-half inches in height. Now he is back to fiftieth percentile for height and about thirty to fortieth percentile for weight. Our doctor said it is more important that he grows taller than gain significant weight.

My husband and I are happy that his appetite improved which increased his growth, stabilized his health and improved his behavior over the past year. Furthermore, the allergy to the egg has improved, falling from a five to a three (on a scale of one to five). The dairy allergy has stabilized and remained at three. We have been giving our second son the same dosage as our first son starting at age two. We started taking the same dosage ourselves as well. The cost of the probiotics is about twenty-five dollars for a month's supply. We keep the probiotics in the refrigerator and are careful to buy the brand that is dairy-free. We feel probiotics are working well for our sons.

Wanting to share the experience and possible benefits, I wrote an article entitled, "Probiotics Help Local Kids with Food Allergies" for the *Boston Parents Paper*, which is reprinted here with permission.[144]

After just five days on probiotics, my three-year-old son said, "I hungry!" for the first time. My husband and I looked at each other with wide eyes. From the day he was born, my son, who is allergic to several different foods, has had trouble recognizing hunger.

After nine months of taking probiotics—bacteria that naturally occurs in food, such as yogurt—we brought him in for a regular food allergy test and discovered that his allergies had improved. His allergy to chicken disappeared, his egg allergy went from severe to moderate and his dairy allergy stabilized at moderate after being "off the charts" for the first two years of his life.

Research into the benefits of probiotics has received plenty of media attention recently, including whether these organisms known to help balance good and bad bacteria in the body can also help prevent food allergies in children. The evidence isn't conclusive, but some families report hopeful results with their own children.

Food allergies currently afflict over eleven million Americans— about four percent of all adults, six to eight percent of school-aged children and eight percent of preschoolers—according to recent statistics gathered by the National Institutes of Allergy and Infectious Diseases and the Asthma and Allergy Foundation of America.

In fact, the incidence of food allergies is on the rise, particularly in children, and no one is sure why. Just ten years ago, scientists believed that less than one percent of the population was affected by a food allergy, according to The Food Allergy & Anaphylaxis Network.[145] But the prevalence of peanut allergies alone doubled from 1997 to 2002, according to a 2003 report in the Journal of Allergy & Clinical Immunology.

Studies have shown that children with a family history of allergies are more likely to suffer allergies themselves. One study even found that children born to women over the age of twenty-nine are about three times more likely to have food allergies, according to the Children's Hospital Boston's Allergy/Immunology program between 1998 and 2000.

Food allergies are different from food intolerances—they're more serious and can result in anaphylactic shock. Ninety percent of these allergies are caused by just eight foods: Dairy, soy, eggs, wheat, peanuts, tree nuts, fish and shellfish. U.S. emergency rooms handle roughly 30,000 allergic reactions each year. Families suffer from about two hundred allergy-related deaths of loved ones each year, according to the Archives of Internal Medicine.

Probiotics primarily help the body maintain a balance of good bacteria, which in turn helps protect us from illness. While bad bacteria in our systems can make us ill, too little of the good can leave us vulnerable to serious illness. When we're sick, antibiotics help destroy the bad bacteria causing our sickness but can also destroy the good bacteria we still need. Probiotics are generally taken to restore the good bacteria. Lactobacillus acidophilus, found in yogurt is a probiotic, as is yeast and the flavored drink *kefir*.

Studies have shown that probiotics can help reduce the risk of certain diarrhea, aid digestion for people with lactose intolerance and improve the body's immune function. But can probiotics help reduce or even prevent food allergies?

Athos Bousvaros, M.D., a pediatric gastro-intestinal specialist at Children's Hospital in Boston, says there is evidence that probiotics may help prevent food allergies in children. Specifically, two recent international studies show a reduction and improvement in eczema (a symptom of a food allergy) when probiotics are administered proactively.

"An important study was done in Finland by Erica Isolauri, where it was shown that probiotics may help with eczema, food allergies and asthma," Bousvaros notes. In the study, a group of pregnant women were given probiotics during their third trimesters and their newborns were given probiotics supplements for the first six months of life. Another group received placebos. The study, published in the medical journal The Lancet in 2001, found that by one year of age, forty-six percent of the placebo group of infants had eczema, compared to only twenty-three percent of the probiotics group.

"The second study focused on treatment," Bousvaros says. Researcher Susan Prescott, M.D., in Australia, conducted a study in 2005 that investigated the effects of probiotics in fifty-three children, ages six months to eighteen months, with moderate or severe atopic dermatitis (eczema). The children were given either a probiotic (lactobacillus fermentum) or a placebo, twice daily for eight weeks. After sixteen weeks, the reduction in the severity of eczema was significant in the probiotic group but not the placebo group.

Still, some researchers acknowledge that studies haven't provided enough evidence. In a scientific review published in The Journal of Allergy and Clinical Immunology, Prescott and fellow researcher Bengt Bjorkstén, M.D., concluded that while the theory that probiotics may reduce or prevent food allergies is "sound," there isn't enough data "to recommend probiotics as a part of standard therapy in any allergic conditions."

Furthermore, in this country, studies are heavily regulated by the National Institutes of Health and can be expensive. "Because the question hasn't been asked enough in the U.S., little funding has been allocated by the government for studies on probiotics and food allergies," Bousvaros says.

Despite a lack of formal studies in the U.S., however, children with food allergies are benefiting from probiotics. Massachusetts mother Haleh has three sons, the youngest boy endures the most severe case of allergies in Haleh's family. He is allergic to peanuts, tree nuts, dairy, soy, egg, oats, wheat and sesame. When her son was about four and one-half, Haleh began religiously giving him a probiotics capsule each evening. "Six months later, at his next food allergy test, his allergies had declined in severity by about fifty percent," Haleh says. "There was additional improvement at his next allergy test at age five and one-half.

The most significant improvement occurred with the egg and dairy allergies," Haleh reports.

Pennsylvania mother Gina's youngest son is allergic to peanuts, tree nuts, seeds, dairy, egg and wheat, as well as some fruits and vegetables. She says his severe symptoms of eczema and his food allergies began to improve after six months on probiotics. Gina even recalls running out of probiotics, neglecting to buy more and then noticing that her son's eczema returned. "I swear by probiotics!" she says.

Probiotics can be obtained through supplements, which look like vitamins and can be purchased at health food stores. They also occur naturally in certain foods, including the following:

Yogurt: A bacterial fermented milk pudding.
Kefir: A Turkish or Mongolian fermented milk drink.
Tempeh: An Indonesian white soybean cake.
Miso: A Japanese rice, barley or soybean paste.
Sauerkraut: A German or Polish cabbage dish.
Kim Chi: A Korean seasoned vegetable dish.

Foods with probiotics supplements include Yacult, a Japanese probiotics milk popular in western Europe since 1950, and Dannon's Activia yogurt which contains bifidus regularis. Beech Nut's Good Evening baby food contains *pre*biotics (not *pro*biotics), which stimulate growth of good bacteria.

"There are normally no negative side effects to taking one to two probiotic supplements a day," Bousvaros says, "Occasionally, a stomachache or diarrhea might emerge, but this is unusual. Probiotic capsules can be broken and put into juice or formula, but shouldn't be heated above body temperature since this could kill the beneficial bacteria. If a child is very sick with an intestinal disorder, then probiotics bacterium could cause bacteria to go into the bloodstream, which would be dangerous."

As with most treatments, parents who are considering giving their allergic child probiotics should consult their physician before doing so. Certainly, it's worth asking about benefits and encouraging more studies on the effects of probiotics on food allergies in the U.S. These allergies may be dubbed "the invisible disability," but a cure might be visible and within reach. {End of reprinted article.}

Social Situations

CHAPTER 43: BIRTHDAY PARTIES

One of the most difficult toddler activities are birthday parties because food is always involved. There can be snacks on a table for all little hands to reach and there can be a lunch or a dinner for everyone to share. There is always a birthday cake that usually contains a host of common allergen ingredients. Sometimes the ingredients are not obvious but can be equally dangerous. A local kindergarten teacher told me about a child who had a reaction to cake because almond extract was used in the frosting. The hidden dangers are the most dangerous.

If the food theme includes a food to which a child is highly allergic then the best response is to decline the invitation to the party. Our allergist advised us that when food is heated the food can go into the air and be inhaled. This can possibly cause a reaction in an allergic child. Therefore, we avoid parties that are centered on a pizza theme because our sons have a dairy allergy. In several cases, once I declined the invitation, the parents readily changed the food theme of the party to something less dangerous for our boys. For instance, hot dogs, hamburgers or sandwiches were served. In other cases, it was not easily feasible to change the food theme, especially if the birthday party was held at a facility that hosted the party. Pizza is an especially difficult item to avoid. It is popular in our country, easy to order and to serve. The danger remains, though, for the children with dairy allergy.

Imagine a child who has a peanut allergy. If invited to a peanut butter and jelly sandwich party, it might seem more obvious to decline the invitation. Similarly, if the party included a treasure hunt for walnuts or hazelnuts then a child with a tree nut allergy would be equally in danger. These examples may seem silly, but it is our experience that foods containing dairy, specifically, are prevalent in our culture and difficult to avoid. Cakes with butter and milk, ice cream popsicles, cones and side dishes are common, cheese puffs, corn chips, fish crackers and cheese or butter crackers are widespread and sour cream dips usually accompany otherwise harmless vegetables.

On the other hand, if the party and food theme do not appear to be overtly dangerous to our boys allergic situation, then we happily attend. There are some precautions that we take. Specifically, I call the mother several days ahead of time and ask what color the cake and frosting will be. For instance, she might have ordered a vanilla cake with chocolate frosting. Sometimes the cake is heavily colored with a theme such as Spiderman red or Batman blue. My goal is to make a cake or a few cup-cakes for my boys to eat while the other kids eat the cake. The allergen-free cake should look as much as possible like the real birthday cake so that we do not draw attention to the fact that our boys have allergies and thus feel different.

One of my personal goals is to make our boys feel normal and part of the group. For that reason, I used to try to sneak the making of the cupcakes and the serving of the cake during the party to my boys. After a few of these attempts, I found it easier and better not to. For one thing it was too hard to make the cake without my older son knowing. He ac-tually really likes helping me in the kitchen and gets excited about the birthday party in part by making the cake for his friend's party. In addi-tion, since he is already familiar with the cake we made, he is less con-fused when served the cake, because he knows it is okay for him to eat it. When I snuck it to him, he inquisitively looked at me for permission to eat the "real" birthday cake. Of course, it was the allergen-free one, so I said, "yes," but trying to pretend it is the real cake doesn't buy us much. The bottom line is that if the other kids don't really notice that our boys' cake is different, then that is what counts, because my sons are happy and feel included.

It is hard to make a cake without using dairy or eggs. But, I found two relatively foolproof recipes: a chocolate cake and a white cake. The chocolate frosting can be used for either. Each of the ingredients below should be closely reviewed to ensure that there are no allergens present or potentially present for your child for his or her specific allergies.

White Cake

3 cups cake flour

1 3/4 cups sugar

1 1/4 cups water

1/2 cup shortening

2 1/2 tsp. baking powder

1 tsp. salt

1 1/2 tsp. vanilla extract

mixed together before adding:

3 tablespoon water, 3 tablespoon canola oil, 2 tsp. baking powder;

Preheat oven to 350 degrees. Grease and flour two cake pans. In a large bowl, combine all ingredients. Using an electric mixer, beat until well mixed, approximately four minutes. Pour batter into cake pans. Bake for 40 to 45 minutes, until cake tester inserted in center comes out clean. Cool in pans ten minutes before removing to wire racks. Frost when completely cooled.[146]

Chocolate Cake

3 cups flour

1 3/4 cups white sugar

2/3 cups cocoa powder

2 tsp. baking soda

1 tsp. salt

2 cups water

2/3 cups vegetable oil

2 tsp. vanilla

2 tsp. white vinegar

Mix first five ingredients together well. Add remaining ingredients and mix well again. Pour into greased and cocoa-ed pan(s) and back at 350 degrees or until a toothpick comes out clean. 13 x 9 pan for 30 to 35 minutes. Cupcakes for 15 minutes. (originally from John's "Chocolate! Chocolate! Chocolate!")

Chocolate Frosting

1/2 cup milk-free, soy-free margarine, softened
1/2 cup unsweetened cocoa powder
2 2/3 cups unsifted confectioners sugar
1/4 cup water
1 tsp. vanilla extract

Beat margarine on medium speed in large mixer bowl until softened, about one minute. Add remaining ingredients. Beat on low speed until ingredients are moistened. Beat on medium speed until creamy. [147]

As for non-cake foods served at the party, there are two options we use. First and foremost, we always bring a few little snack bags of our own safe snacks so that if the second option fails, we have something to give to our children. The second option is to check out the ingredient labels of the snacks being served. Normally, the bags are on the counter in the kitchen or if hosted at a third party location, the snacks might be in a brown paper bag brought by the parents. I usually simply ask the parent, "Do you mind if I look at the ingredients of the pretzels (and other snacks)?" No one ever seems to mind. Then, once I have ascertained which party snacks are safe, I'll quickly prepare a plate for each of my children ahead of time so there is no confusion if they try to go to the snack table during the "rush."

With respect to drinks, juice boxes seem to be a popular solution for most parties. I have found that these juice drinks often have natural or artificial flavors or are supplemented with a calcium product that is derived from dairy. Therefore, I often do not feel comfortable giving my sons the juice box. For this reason, I try to have some juice boxes on hand at home that I can throw in the snack bag to bring along. If I fail to do this, the result is not pretty. My sons do feel left out and become unruly if I try to give them water or their sippy cups with juice or cider from home. The only salvation is that normally bottled water might suffice since drinking from the bottle is a novelty.

Another tricky problem is when ice pops are served. Again, most fruit ice pops actually contain dairy. In these cases, I have made our ice pops at home in a plastic ice pop container with juice that I know is safe. Transporting the ice pops requires a cooler. Since I don't like to put them in the freezer of the host, since the freezer usually contains ice creams drips and drops, keeping the ice pops cold is difficult at best. Fortunately, ice pops are relatively uncommon at the birthday parties that we have attended.

Finally, the last difficulty with birthday parties is the goody bag handed out at the end of the party. Some of my friends will actually prepare a couple of food-free goody bags for my children and mark them with a special, yet inconspicuous, sticker. This is so thoughtful of them for which I always feel grateful. In some cases, I've managed to bring a little allergen-free candy from home to slip into the bags for my sons. In other cases, I must remove the candy from the bags before letting my children have them. Since these bags are given out on the way out of the party, this issue is normally easily handled quickly in the car or at home. Further the children are usually so excited and tired that they don't seem to notice or care too much.

CHAPTER 44: TODDLER ACTIVITIES

While birthday parties are difficult, the good news is that other toddler activities can be relatively easy, if chosen carefully. For instance, gymnastic classes are usually forty-five minute classes in which food is nowhere in sight. In fact it would be unsafe for the children to be eating while jumping around and swinging on gymnastic equipment. Another good choice is swimming lessons or free swim. Food normally is not present at organized swim class or free swim. There was one occasion where the swim teacher handed out chocolate filled lollipops after the last class of the session. Since the chocolate center of these lollipops contains dairy, my son could not have one. Had I known she was going to do this, I'd have brought a lollipop for my son. But the best I had on hand was a banana. My son wasn't impressed with the banana. In that case, I had to simply tell my son, "I am sorry but you are allergic to those lollipops. I'll give you a lollipop when we get home." Once I said that, he understood and handled it pretty well.

We love to go to the library. It is great fun for the children and cost effective (free). At first I was skeptical about taking my noisy children here but I found there was an entire floor dedicated to children and it wasn't that quiet. There was a playroom filled with toys including a train table and puzzles. The local public library in our area also offers some free programs for toddlers and preschoolers. They have classes listed on a hand out on the librarians' desk and also on the Internet. The boys love the classes in which the librarian reads a few stories then gives them a small art project and finishes up by singing a few songs. It lasts forty-five minutes. We then go up to the playroom for an hour or so. The kids just love it.

When we signed up for the library class, there was a line to indicate whether there were food allergies. I did indicate that our children had allergies. I believe they might have handed out a snack otherwise. Another concern might be that an art project might include some food, for instance, making something out of an egg carton. We would definitely avoid that project. Or, the art project might include gluing dry noodles onto some paper. That project would be fine, unless the noodles were egg noodles.

Another favorite activity is going to indoor playgrounds. About ten miles away is an indoor playground. The cost is about eight dollars per child to play all day, from ten o'clock to three o'clock. No food is allowed in the play area and there are signs all around saying, "Absolutely No Food or Drink Allowed." The play area consists of air jumping rooms, slides, a big netted jungle gym, a trolley, a basketball net, little houses and a sandbox. The room appears to be about six thousand square feet and is clean. There is a separate area for eating in an adjacent room.

When we take a break to eat, I select a picnic table that is a bit more remote and looks clean. I then wipe it with a disinfectant wipe, not just a diaper wipe. I make sure to wipe the edge of the table since my children seem to touch the edge a lot and have even licked the edge of the table, much to my dismay. I also wipe my boys' hands with a diaper wipe or better yet sometimes take them into the restroom and wash their hands in the sink. After we eat, I wipe the boys' hands again so we don't bring any trace foods back into the play area in case other children have allergies to items we just ate. This effort feels good and is the right thing to do. I hope people don't bring foods like peanut butter to places like this for the sake of the children who have peanut allergies, since these allergies are so severe and the trace is so difficult to remove from the environment. There are options, such as soy nut butter which tastes almost the same as peanut butter.

Outdoor playgrounds offer a slightly more difficult challenge since the area is not supervised and parents allow their children to bring food onto the slides and other play things. As I watch my children, I will scan the other children for food or drinks. There have been times when I have asked parents not to let their children eat on the apparatus and explain that my children have food allergies. I don't apologize, but I don't get angry either. I try to be as matter-of-fact about it as possible.

For instance, once we were at a park when there were three girls eating a bag of cookies at the top of the platform for a large slide. They had the entire bag of cookies up there. I was concerned that my sons might be given a cookie or that they'd be touching the crumbs of the cookie and accidentally get some into their mouths or even onto their skin. There is a conflict that emerges inside of me when confronted with this situation. On the one hand, I have been taught to be polite and mind my own business to a certain degree. To step outside of that space and actually tell someone else how I feel or what I'd like him or her to do, is uncomfortable to say the least. I tell myself that my child's health is at stake, this is my *job* to protect my child, and that I don't have to be angry with the people, just straightforward. These thoughts help me deal with the situation. This time I said, "My children have food allergies and I think your children have a bag of cookies at the top of the slide." On this occasion it went well. The other mom called to her daughter to bring the cookies down. She smiled and said she was sorry. I smiled and responded, "Thank you."

At other times it can be slightly less smooth. On a different day, a mother was letting her young daughter, possibly two or three years of age, eat a sandwich on the equipment. I was thinking the sandwich might fall apart and the insides would open up and get smeared onto the equipment. Not only was I concerned about mayonnaise (egg based) coming in contact with my sons for allergy reasons, but for cleanliness reasons as well. I thought it was rude to let a child walk around up on the equipment with something that could make such a big mess. I said to the other mom, "My sons are allergic to eggs and I noticed your daughter was walking around with a sandwich on the equipment." Her less then helpful response was something like, "It is just a ham sandwich with mayonnaise." So I repeated my concern by saying, "Yes, we have an egg allergy." Again she did not easily comprehend my concern. In fact, I think she may not have realized that mayonnaise is made primarily of eggs. Then her friend seemed to have quietly said this to her because she changed her attitude and retrieved the sandwich from her daughter. Again, I smiled and said, "Thank you, I really appreciate it."

I think the most important part of expressing a concern about food being carried about at a park is not to express the annoyance that I might be feeling. Instead, I try to be matter-of-fact about my children's food allergies. Although I might be feeling anger or frustration, I think the base feeling is fear—simply being afraid that something bad might happen to my children. I always try to thank people and smile.

Another area of concern for outdoor playgrounds is the litter on the ground. Unfortunately my children love to pick up litter, so I have to dash over and get there first. One time there was a buttery bagel discarded on the grass. I didn't see it, but my two-year-old son did. He picked it up and brought it to me. This did not make me happy. I immediately wiped his hands. Interestingly, I was acquainted with the mother whose child had been eating it. I indeed felt highly annoyed that time and am sure this came across, however unfortunate. She called over to say that she was sorry. I feel that it is just plain sloppy and inconsiderate to allow your child to throw food onto the ground. That has not happened often. But discarded drink containers and food wrappers are more prevalent, especially for granola bars, which usually contain peanuts. Normally, when I first arrive at a playground, I scan the ground and jungle-gyms. I pick up and toss wrappers and containers in the trash—I don't like doing this. Then I'll wipe my hands and use the liquid gel cleanser to remove trace allergens and germs off of my own hands.

Another activity to consider is a music class. There are mommy and me groups that meet to sing songs and play with musical toys. We never actually took any of these classes since my boys were so active and I didn't feel they'd sit still long enough. But perhaps they would have. At any rate, this type of class probably will not involve food especially if the teacher is notified of your child's food allergies.

Another activity that we do, as I am sure everyone does, is watch television and videos. I only allow our boys to watch a few stations that do not have commercials and that do not show violent cartoons. Public television and television geared towards toddlers is best. We occasionally watch an animal station as well but not if the animals are eating each other. We watch movies and educational videos as well. I cannot overstate how valuable the educational videos have become. I recently purchased several videos on learning letters and reading, as well as numbers and basic math. My husband and I were pleasantly surprised to see how the children learned their letters, letter sounds and reading concepts from these videos. The children love the videos and want to watch them repeatedly for weeks at a time. I ordered these videos over the Internet and was able to find them for between five and twelve dollars each. This money was well spent. When they are watching these videos, I feel good about them watching television. Otherwise, I feel that they are wasting their time.

Reading books is an excellent activity for toddlers. I have found that the television needs to be turned off for this to be successful, otherwise they are too distracted. We read to our children every night before bed. I try to read with them during the day as well. There are some books at the library that help children learn kindergarten skills such as simple math, counting, letters and maps readings. I recently read an article which advised that the more books are in a home, the brighter the children tend to be.

One final note, sometimes there are activities that involve food, such as Halloween in which we participate. Depending upon the sensitivity of your child's allergies, there might be safe ways to allow your child to participate. Specifically, for Halloween, when our son was about three, we took him trick-or-treating, but *we* put the candy into the pumpkin-shaped bag for him. This past year, we considered putting gloves on his hands, but decided to allow him to put the candy into the bag himself. We did not let him eat any candy and washed his hands when we got back to the car. When we arrived home, I had prepared a separate pumpkin tin of candy for each of our boys filled with candy that I had purchased from the health food store which had no egg, dairy, peanut or tree nut trace in it. One of their favorite candies is the one hundred percent pure maple syrup sugar candies. They were thrilled and ate their favorite and new candy happily. I took all of the candy from trick-or-treating and tossed it into the trash in the garage. Although we allow our sons to trick-or-treat, we avoid Halloween parties. At a party there would be a lot of trace allergens on the other children's hands from eating the candy.

In summary, finding activities for your food-allergic child can be done in a way that reduces the likelihood of coming into contact with allergens. Look in the phonebook, newspaper, library and church walls for activities. Call the Parks and Recreation Department in your local town for their schedule of activities. I found our best activities were at a gym, pool or library and going to the playgrounds. Always bring plenty of allergen-free food from home.

CHAPTER 45: FRIENDS AND PLAY DATES

Although we were willing to give up allergen-foods, we were not willing to give up friends for ourselves and our children. We did not want to feel isolated. We value our friendships. Therefore, we make efforts to have friends over, to visit or meet at public places several times a week. Some friends found it easier than others to eliminate food allergens during play dates. Specifically, some friends would ask, "What kinds of snacks can I put out that are okay for your kids?" I would respond, "Fresh fruits, vegetables, potato chips and pretzels." For the chips and pretzels, I would add the brand name and the flavor. I.e. for the chips I would say, plain, non-flavored in the yellow bag of brand X. My friends were appreciative of this information and they felt good to provide safe food for the children to eat while they played. I recommend that if someone asks you what your kids can eat, be straightforward about it and specific. It is just a problem that needs to be solved.

Some friends found it too overwhelming to cater to our needs or to eliminate food entirely from a play date. Their children would grow hungry within the hour and needed to eat. Otherwise, their children would get cranky. Without a little planning ahead, the situation becomes difficult as the mother rifles through her refrigerator that seems to be filled with nothing other than dairy products. For these friends, we'd either try to meet at a public place such as a park, or I'd try to maintain my friendship through email, telephone or adult dinners.

In contrast, some friends understood allergies so well that I trusted them enough to leave my children with them. For instance, we needed to leave our son with friends when I was in labor with our second son. The friends we called had experience with two older children who had some allergies. Plus they had seen our son react to dairy one time. They were shocked at how quickly and severely the hives had appeared on my son's face. We felt wholly comfortable leaving our son with them.

When we have dinner parties, we were always sure to serve allergen-free foods in our home. This was easy to do since we were already fully entrenched in an allergen-free diet and could prepare foods that tasted good. For instance, I would prepare meals such as steak with baked potatoes and salad with dressing that did not contain cheese or milk. Usually balsamic vinaigrette would work well and most people like this kind of dressing. Another favorite was preparing a beef roast with roasted rosemary potatoes and cauliflower. We also liked to serve barbequed pork spare ribs with whole grain rice and broccoli. Most of these things were easy to cook so that time could be spent with friends rather than cooking in the kitchen.

Friends always like to bring something to the dinner. It was difficult for some of them not to bring something, even when asked not to. So again, I'd let them know what did work for us that they could bring. Specifically, I might suggest a vegetable salad (with no dressing), or a fresh fruit salad. Or most people seemed perfectly happy to bring some wine or beer. I learned that I needed to ask what their children liked to eat to avoid their bringing foods into our home which contained dairy. Their children were more likely to be happy with the foods we offered if planning was done ahead of time.

When we go to a friend's house for dinner there are two options. We can either discuss the menu with our friends beforehand to select foods that work for the children, or we can bring our own food for the children. If we bring our own food, we just pop it in the microwave at dinner time and can probably serve an item or two from the hostess' menu as well. We ask that they avoid foods heavy in cheese, especially hot cheese, since our allergist advised that hot cheese actually goes into the air and may trigger and allergic reaction. For this reason we outright decline gatherings that will include pizza. If your child has a peanut or tree nut allergy, don't be shy about requesting these foods are not placed on the table as a snack or appetizer. The same goes for seafood or fish—ask for a fish-free environment.

If it is too difficult to have a food-friendly play date, then another option is to set up a play date at a public location. Play dates can be held at libraries, indoor playgrounds, outdoor playgrounds, children's museums, zoos, or walking trails. Sometimes signing children up for the same music or gymnastics class can be a fun and educational way to get the children together.

CHAPTER 46: PRESCHOOL—IS IT WORTH IT?

It seems that most people we know send their children to preschool. Some start as early as two years, others wait until three years, so the children have between two and three years of preschool under their belts prior to entering kindergarten. Most children go to two or three days of preschool for two to four hours. Some children go to preschool four days or five days a week for four hours each day. The skills that my friends say they want their children to develop mostly include socialization skills, writing letters and learning numbers.

When you consider preschool, I recommend researching several preschools' policies and interviewing staff members. Get recommendations from friends and those who have had their children attend the preschools that you are considering. Many preschools are open to allowing prospective attendees to watch a session—take advantage and observe a session. Also ask your pediatrician and allergist for his or her opinion about preschool for your child with his or her specific situation. Ultimately I believe the most important concern at this stage is safety. It is up to the parents to protect their child, since the child is too young to fully understand his or her allergies and the ramifications. Do what is best for your child within their particular situation and your available options.

We opted not to send our children to preschool. The primary reason was because of food allergies. Specifically, we did not want to expose our children to either an accidental dose of dairy (which is found in most prepackaged foods) or trace amounts of dairy from the other children's snacks and hands. Our allergist told us at our first appointment that the best chance a child has for outgrowing a dairy allergy is to avoid it completely. She later told us about an incident in which a child who is allergic to dairy was at a daycare when a pizza party was being held. The daycare providers placed the child in a high chair so he would not touch the pizza. Even so, the child had a reaction because the cheese was heated and went into the air. The child broke out in hives just by smelling the pizza.

Another consideration was the trace amounts of allergens on the toys from the other children's hands. We felt that any environment that allowed food would be an increased risk for our children. Although we encourage our children to play with other children in public places and at their homes, it is under our supervision to be sure there are no foods heavy in dairy protein, such as nacho-cheese corn chips, which have a tendency to leave a lot of residue on fingertips. There would be no way to make this determination at a preschool environment because we would not be there to supervise.

I became concerned about our decision not to send our children to preschool. Would they have the skills they needed upon entering kindergarten in the immediate future? What were the short-term and long-term impacts? After doing some research I was surprised at what I found. I found the short, medium and long-term benefits of preschool might not be as high as often touted.

It has been found that the short-term impact of preschool on children is an increase in stress level and poor behavior. For example, one study found that cortisol, a stress hormone, was *raised* in children when they spent time away from home. The more time away from home, the more stress hormone was found in their bodies.[148] Another study found that both teachers and mothers agreed that the behavior of their preschooler was hindered by preschool, not helped. Specifically, according to Stanford, University of California, and National Institute of Child Health and Human Development, "We find that attendance in preschool centers, even for short periods of time each week, hinders the rate at which young children develop social skills and display the motivation to engage classroom tasks, as reported by their kindergarten teachers....We might guess that the problem lies with poor quality preschool centers. But even high income children—who presumably attend the better preschools—showed increased behavioral problems if they had attended at least fifteen hours a week...The more time children spend in centers, the worse their behavior becomes...Researchers found that the more time children spent in non-maternal care during the first four and one-half years of life, the more behavioral problems they developed. Problems included defiance—like talking back, throwing temper tantrums and refusing to cooperate. They also included aggressive behaviors—being cruel, destroying toys and other objects and getting into physical fights. In addition, kids who spent more time in childcare were rated as less socially competent by their mothers and kindergarten teachers."[149]

While there appear to be negative effects on social skills, are there positive effects on academic skills? Would my children be behind in their development? I found a study that indicated a leveling effect over the first couple of years in school where a University of California study states, "By the end of third grade, according to Rumberger's research, former preschoolers and children who did not attend preschool ended up on nearly equal footing in cognitive and social development..."[150]

Finally, any hoped-for long-term positive impact of preschool on children hasn't been found either. According to the CATO Institute, "The arguments in favor of preschool education were that it would reduce school failure, lower dropout rates, increase test scores, and produce a generation of more competent high school graduates...Preschool education will achieve none of these results."[151] The Reason Foundation appears to concur stating, "The Rand study actually cites evidence...showing that middle and upper-income kids get no long-term gain from preschool participation."[152]

I have often felt social pressure to enroll our sons in preschool. I know of only two other mothers who decided not to send their children to preschool. One said she believes, "It's a scam." I have heard that about ninety percent of children attend preschool prior to entering kindergarten, so there is a lot of peer pressure on parents. Another mother told me, "I wasn't going to send my son to preschool, but all of his friends were there, so we did." Because of this pressure, I reminded myself, as did my husband, many times over the years of the risks associated with our sons' food allergies along with the lack of evidence showing the benefits of preschool. Instead, we invested in purchasing workbooks, educational videos, art supplies and other educational items for our sons while with placing the preschool cost savings into college education savings.

While we decided that preschool wasn't for us, I can understand that a parent might not be willing to give up preschool. For instance a mother might want or need a break from watching and teaching the children. Or she might feel that she doesn't have the patience to teach the basic skills of reading, writing, numbers and math. Or a mother of an "only-child" might find it challenging to expose her child to others regularly. She may worry about her child's social development with peers. Another consideration is that a mother may feel overly anxious or even paranoid about bringing her child into new environments where the food situation is unknown. For all of those reasons, preschool can remain an option if a safe environment can be found. Many preschools offer an allergen-free environment especially for peanuts and tree nuts. I haven't encountered any preschools that guarantee an allergen-free environment for dairy, egg, soy, wheat, fish or shellfish. I think dairy, soy and wheat are most difficult to avoid, especially since many snack foods contain at least two of these ingredients.

I have discussed the risks versus benefits of preschool with a friend of mine who is a first-grade teacher. During that discussion, I explained the skills that we are teaching our children at home. She replied, "It sounds like you are teaching your children a lot of skills and your children should be fine in kindergarten. The risks of the allergies versus benefits of preschool are clearly not worth it in your case." This provided me with the extra assurance I wanted. My son will enter kindergarten in the coming year. It will be interesting to see how he does.

Whenever faced with decisions such as whether or not to send our children to preschool, I like to learn more about what is involved and to make an educated choice. For this reason, I thought about and researched what is involved in "home-schooling" our preschoolers. Both social and academic skills are explored in the following chapter, with the hope that it will help you make a decision that is best for you and your children.

CHAPTER 47: KINDERGARTEN READINESS

Once we made the decision to keep our children out of preschool, I began to research what skills they will need upon entering kindergarten. My research is based upon talking with friends, attending pre-kindergarten discussion groups, talking with grammar school teachers, reading and research. Based upon that research, preschoolers should be acquainted with letters, reading, writing, drawing shapes, numbers and basic math. They should also be trained in following instructions, taking turns, sharing and resolving conflicts in non-aggressive ways.

My husband and I have purchased DVDs on the alphabet, learning to read, counting and basic math. Our boys love to watch these DVDs over and over. We were pleasantly surprised at how quickly they learned skills like the sounds letters make and counting by tens. We also work with our sons to teach them writing and drawing. We found they started by using templates to help them draw the letters by tracing in the holes. We do some of our work like writing at the kitchen table and reading before bed, but have discovered that lessons also work well in non-traditional environments, such as in the car or at the park. For instance, while my sons are playing on the jungle-gyms, I will say, "What is two plus two?" My older son will grumble for a second but then shout out, "Four!" Both boys see who can answer the questions faster. We also count things like the steps on the ladder. Sometimes we'll play store at the park and pretend to exchange quarters, dimes, nickels and pennies.

In addition to the tangible skills of letters and numbers, my husband and I make a special effort to teach the boys social skills of following instructions, taking turns, sharing and resolving conflicts. For instance, by going to library classes, swimming classes and soccer camp they have successfully learned to listen to a teacher and participate in the class by taking turns with the other children. I also give them instructions to follow at home. For instance, I might ask them to pick up an object from the floor. I'll describe where the object is and point to it. Even though it might be faster for me to pick it up, I'd take the extra time to instruct them. It was often quite challenging for them to find the object at which I was pointing, just a few feet away, in plain sight. Eventually, they became good at this little game. I'd also ask them to do little tasks such as carry their own diaper to the garbage or go get a spoon out of the silverware drawer. This gave them the opportunity to listen, remember and execute the instruction. I have watched my husband do the same. We are always careful to praise them as well.

I have also tried to teach our children to share. Since our children are close in age (nineteen months apart) and the same sex (boys), they are constantly challenged by sharing toys with one another. When they have a dispute with each other that isn't too serious, I try not to intervene. I want to allow them to work it out. I've even noticed that their conflicts are usually less severe when they think I am not watching. I've noticed that once they see me, sometimes the conflicts escalate. It must be to get my attention—sometimes they look to me to resolve their conflict. I like the fact that when they think I am not around, they are able to resolve most issues without conflict. When friends are involved, sharing is reasonably well done. But, I have noticed they have a little more trouble sharing toys with children with whom they are not well acquainted. To challenge them with sharing, we have play dates and visit the playroom at the library. They also spend time in the food-free child-watch room at the health club that is filled with toys. I normally ask how our children behaved during the stay. Most of the time the report is good, and when there has been an issue, it is usually between our own children.

When conflicts do arise, I believe they should be resolved in a non-aggressive way. Unfortunately, it seems that the natural way children handle conflicts is to push, hit, bite or any number of other undesirable behaviors. So my husband and I try to teach our children to walk away from someone who is bothering them or take a break and a deep breath.

I hope that if another child tries to push food that contains allergens onto our children, they can walk away. I have sat with my older son and worked with him on this issue. Specifically, I say, "What would you say if someone at school says, 'Here, eat this—it is really good'?" My son responds, "I would say, 'No thank-you, I have allergies,'" and he puts his hand up like a traffic-cop to accentuate the point. I praise him and explain to him how people might not understand how dairy can be found in a cracker, cookie or piece of bread—and that is okay as long as he walks away. It isn't his job to convince them that the cookie has dairy in it.

If you decide to "home-school" your preschooler, you should research the skills that your state recommends. For example, our state's Department of Education publishes the following pamphlet entitled, "Getting Your Child Ready for Kindergarten."[153] I thought I would reprint them here.

Skills for Speaking and Listening:

- *Use and understand many words:* Use new words daily as you play together and go about everyday activities. For example, "I am going to a mechanic to have my car fixed."

- *Speak in complete sentences:* Be a model for your child by speaking in complete sentences with five or more words per sentence. Help your child to add words to complete his or her sentences.

- *Ask lots of questions:* Listen carefully to your child's questions, and together spend time to find out the answers.

- *Say and notice words that rhyme in stories:* Say and sing nursery rhymes, rap and poetry, and play rhyme games. Help him or her to repeat the words that rhyme. Help your child to make up his or her own funny rhyming words.

- *Make up and share personal stories about his or her interests:* Listen with interest to your child's stories, make comments and ask questions. Share your own stories. Show your own childhood photographs and tell stories about them.

Skills for Reading and Writing:

- *Select familiar books and tell why he or she likes them:* Retell favorite stories from books: Take your child to the library to select books. Read with your child and discuss things that your child likes about the books.

- *Hold a book upright:* Read books that your child likes over and over. Read books often with your child so he or she learns how to hold and use a book. Allow your child to pretend to "read" to you favorite stories from books.

- *Identify letters of the alphabet:* Have your child point out and say the letters in his or her name; put magnetic letters of the alphabet on the refrigerator for your child to use. Help your child to point out letters on cereal boxes, street signs and stores.

- *Recognize letter sounds:* Introduce your child to the sounds of letters by helping your child to say the sound of the first letter of his or her name. Have your child find or say things that begin with the same letter sound of his or her name. Have your child say the sounds of the first letters of the names of his or her brothers and sisters, and sounds of letters that your child is interested in.

- *Recognize, copy and print his or her first name:* Print your child's name whenever possible, such as on his or her drawings or below his or her photograph. Provide pencils, crayons or markers and paper for your child to scribble or write his or her first name. Help your child recognize shapes in letters that form his or her name.

- *Hold a pencil and write with it*: Let your child see you writing for various reasons, such as making a shopping list or writing a birthday card. Provide pencils, crayons or markers and paper for your child to make marks, scribble or write in his or her own way.

Mathematic Skills:

- *Recognize and count up to ten items:* Turn meal times into counting fun by having your child count objects as he or she helps set the table. Count objects whenever you are driving or walking to school or on errands. Check out the local library for counting books—children love to read and re-read these books.

- *Recognize the number symbols 1-10:* Play "I Spy" with numbers as you travel; find numbers in books; count, measure and estimate while making dinner. Look for number symbols in magazines, cut out and glue on paper all the 2s, 3s, etc. Put magnetic numbers on the refrigerator for your child to use.

- *Describe and talk about objects that have different sizes, colors, shapes and patterns:* Use a favorite story/picture book—describe objects according to color, shape and size. Play games with dancing and moving to a pattern: hop, wiggle, spin; hop, wiggle, spin. Play guessing games: "Can you find something that is red and round or looks like a triangle?"

- *Color and draw patterns together.*

- *Sort items by "same" and "different":* Play games in which your child has to find the matching sock, shoe and mitten. Set the table by matching every plate with a napkin, cup and fork. Look for picture games, playing cards and dominoes for finding matches.

- *Use the words "near," "far," "top," "bottom," "under," "first," "second," "last":* Use your morning routine to practice "First we get up, second we wash our face." Use the tune of a familiar song to create a movement song: "Put your hands on top of your head;

stand on top of the box; crawl under the table." Use these words in directions: "Put your sneakers under the bed; put the teddy bear on top of the pillow."

- *Sort objects from smallest to largest, shortest to tallest and lightest to heaviest:* Gather a variety of objects from your child's toy box and line them up from largest to smallest. Organize boxes of cereal, rice and pasta from tallest to shortest. Put a variety of objects in a bag; sort them from heaviest to lightest.

Skills for Participation and Cooperation:

- *Understand and participate in conversations:* Set a good example for your child by listening to his or her stories. Encourage your child to tell you about what he or she did during the day.

- *Stay involved in a directed activity to its completion:* Help your child learn to stay with an activity to completion by sharing and working on the activity with him or her. Use positive words of encouragement such as, "You are doing a good job picking up your socks."

- *Follow routines and directions:* Be clear when giving direction to your child. Have your child repeat the directions in his or her own words so you can be sure that he or she understands. Play games with your child such as, "First find the red truck and then the yellow block. Put them both under the blue box." Children may need help in remembering, so remind them by going over the directions.

- *Work and play together with other children:* Provide lots of opportunities for your child to play and participate in groups with other children. Praise your child's efforts and accomplishments. Help your child in solving problems by helping him or her to look at other ways to do something or by giving him or her the words to resolve a conflict.

CHAPTER 48: SCHOOL EMERGENCY PLANS

In determining what type of emergency plan to create for your child upon his or her entering kindergarten, there are two main options. The more serious option is called a 504 Plan. For instance, if the child has a severe reaction to food(s) such as anaphylaxis then the 504 Plan may be in order. The other option is to create an individualized Action Plan. The action plan would provide instructions as to what medication or action to take. The plan that is suitable for a child may change over time. Specifically, as the child grows older, his ability to read labels and monitor his own food intake might dictate that he should be given more freedom. Further, his allergies might decline as he grows older, depending upon the foods to which he is allergic.

"An important goal of the Office for Civil Rights (OCR) is to foster partnerships between school districts and parents to address the needs of students with disabilities. Such partnerships empower all parties to secure quality education. OCR has experienced a steady influx of complaints and inquiries in the area of elementary and secondary education involving Section 504 of the Rehabilitation Act of 1973, as amended, 29 U.S.C. §794 (Section 504). Most of these concern the identification of students who are protected by Section 504 and the means to obtain an appropriate education for such students. OCR reached out to parents and school districts to determine the kinds of assistance they needed."[154] In summary, the Section 504 Plan may be in order for an elementary student who could have an anaphylactic response to eating a food and thereby require medication.

There are arguments for and against having a 504 Plan for your child. The following arguments are from an article entitled, "Food Allergies in Schools: Do You Need a 504 Plan for a Food Allergy?" by Victoria Groce reprinted here with permission.[155]

Arguments for a 504 Plan:

- 504 Plans can be enforced in court, or with the United States Office of Civil Rights, giving your child and family a measure of protection you wouldn't have otherwise had.

- 504 Plans can provide clear guidance for handling your child's allergies even after teachers and staff change in your child's school.

- 504 Plans can address your child's food allergy needs beyond the classroom and in a wide variety of situations more informal discussions might not cover. The evaluation process can help clarify situations—fire drills, field trips, etc.—that might have been overlooked in a less formal talk with teachers.

- Having a written plan and physician authorization may be required in some districts or jurisdictions for students to carry injectible epinephrine on their person.

Arguments against a 504 Plan:

- Obtaining a 504 Plan will be time consuming. An evaluation and assessment of your child is required by statute, and you will need to meet—likely multiple times—with personnel from your child's school (and, potentially, school district) to hammer out plan details. The process may be especially grueling if your school district has never dealt with this issue before.

- If you decide to hire a lawyer to represent your child's interests in crafting a 504 Plan with your school district, or in appealing a denial of a request for a 504 Plan, you may incur substantial legal fees. (You are not required to hire an attorney when creating a 504 Plan—many parents do not.)

- Some parents are concerned about their child "sticking out" due to food allergies. Also, the sheer number of people— administrators, medical personnel, food service personnel, and district compliance officers—who may be involved in developing a 504 Plan can be disconcerting, especially if parents feel their children are close to being able to handle their dietary restrictions independently.

Ms. Groce's article refers to a sample outline for a 504 Plan that was created by a parent and posted by the Food Allergy Initiative.[156] The plan is long, so is not included here fully but rather only the table of contents. Please see the end note above for a reference to the complete plan on the Internet.

SECTION 504 PLAN FOR CHILDREN WITH SEVERE FOOD ALLERGIES

Part A: Student Information
Part B: 504 Team Members and Meeting Information
Part C: Background Information
Part D: Overview of Child's Condition as it Pertains to Section 504
Part E: Goals of the 504 Plan
Part F: Food Allergy Education, Awareness & Reaction Prevention
Part G: Individualized Health Care Plan (IHP)
- Emergency Health Care Plan (EHP)
- Severe Food Allergy Alert Flyer and Emergency Instructions
- Medicine Pack Content List and Location
- Training Documentation
- Student Level of Self-Care Assessment Data Sheet
- Parental Notification of all Allergic Reactions
- Brief Medical History
Part H: Classroom Management
Part I: Instructional Aids
Part J: Substitute Teachers and Nurses
Part K: Bus Transportation
Part L: Signature Page
Part M: Copy of Section 504 of the Rehabilitation Act of 1973 & Copy of Statement of Parental Rights under Section 504
Part N: Additional Resources

If a parent and the school feel that the child does not need a 504 Plan, then informal discussions might suffice. In those cases, an Action Plan may still be provided to the school giving instructions on how to handle a food reaction. The formatting has been removed for the purposes of printing in the book, so be sure to refer to the end note to find the Internet web site that contains the colorful poster that you can provide to your child's school.[157]

ACTION PLAN FOR ANAPHYLAXIS (NON-504)

Name: _____

Date of birth: _____

Photo: _____

Known severe allergies: _____

Parent names: _____

Work phone: _____

Home phone: _____

Cell phone: _____

Known Exposure:
- Spit out the food, if possible
- No symptoms yet
- Give _____ of antihistamine immediately
- Get the EpiPen® Jr. ready in case needed
- Call the parents immediately
- Prepare to call an ambulance

Mild to Moderate Allergic Reaction:
- Swelling of lips, face, eyes
- Hives or welts
- Abdominal pain, vomiting
- Trouble breathing

Watch for signs of Anaphylaxis (Severe Allergic Reaction):
- Difficulty/noisy breathing
- Swelling of tongue
- Swelling/tightness in throat
- Difficulty talking and/or hoarse voice

- Wheeze or persistent cough
- Loss of consciousness and/or collapse
- Pale and floppy (young children)

Action:

- Give EpiPen® Jr. (or EpiPen®), according to doctor's instructions
    1. Form fist around EpiPen® Jr. and pull off grey cap
    2. Place black end against outer mid-thigh
    3. Push down HARD until a click is heard or felt and hold in place for *thirty* seconds
    4. Remove EpiPen® Jr. and be careful not to touch the needle.
    5. Massage the injection site for ten seconds
- Call ambulance. Telephone 911
- Contact parents
- Additional instructions (if necessary)

Plan prepared by:

Dr. _____

Signed _____

Dated _____

Whichever plan you decide to prepare, the most important thing is that the teachers and other people responsible for your child are clear about the foods to which your child is allergic and the potential reactions he or she may have to those foods. This information along with the appropriate medications (EpiPen® Jr., antihistamine and/or asthma inhalers) are imperative for the safety of your child. A periodic check on the information can serve as a valuable reminder to those in charge of your child. I suggest calling the teacher periodically, perhaps once a month, to inquire whether there are any new caretakers (i.e. teacher assistance, substitute teachers, nurses or administrative personnel).

If there is a new caretaker, then request the teacher to explain your child's allergies to the new caretaker or set up a meeting between you and the new caretaker. Follow up with the caretaker after a week or so to see if they have any questions. There are only about nine months to the school year, so making nine telephone calls to inquire and remind those caring for your child is not unreasonable. If the teacher expresses any annoyance, then try to make him or her understand how the life of your child is important to you and that is why you are calling. Furthermore, if he or she is not providing you with a satisfactory sense of safety or new caretaker information, then contact the administrators of the school. There is no need to become aggressive or angry. Kindness and persistence can often be more effective in the long run.

Tricia Dannenhoffer is a first grade teacher and mother of one. Prior to teaching first grade, Ms. Dannenhoffer was an enrichment teacher and coordinator for an elementary school. She has a BA in history, an Elementary Education Certificate and a Masters of Arts in educational psychology with a focus in gifted and talented children. She has been teaching for ten years.

Ms. Dannenhoffer has seen a rise in the incidence of food allergies during her teaching years. She states, "I have definitely seen a rise in the incidence of food allergies. Both the percentage of children with food allergies has risen and the severity has increased significantly as well." In contrast, she points out, "Twenty years ago, when I was attending elementary school, I do not recall any incidence of food allergies. My brother had severe seasonal allergies growing up and that was considered significant in that day and age. But now, seasonal allergies fall to the wayside in a classroom setting because the severity of food allergies has taken precedence."

Ms. Dannenhoffer believes the food allergies can be handled in a variety of ways, and children are adaptable to the behavior that is modeled for them. She explains, "In my classroom, I have a family approach. All students are responsible for looking out for each other's best interest as if they are siblings. We read books and watch educational videos on food allergies. Students then know what their responsibilities are as part of the class. If students understand the significance of food allergies, then they are extremely appropriate and helpful. Again, the students' attitudes depend greatly on the teacher's and other adult attitudes."

Ms. Dannenhoffer states that dealing with food allergies is now part of a teacher's job. For instance, during lunch the teacher or nurse will supervise the peanut-free table in the cafeteria. She describes, "The school nurse and I check each child's lunch box to make sure that there are no peanut or nut ingredients so that friends of the child with allergies can join them for lunch at the peanut-free table. The child with allergies can pick a buddy with whom to eat. This helps the children with allergies feel supported and less different. In fact, it becomes quite the popular thing in my class and kids jump at the chance to join the nut-free table. I have even had parents of children without allergies call because their children insisted on nut-free lunches so they could sit with their friends. For the most part, parents are very helpful and supportive but they need to be as informed as possible."

Positive experiences such as this are excellent. But as with most situations in life, there can be negative influences which produce negative attitudes. Ms. Dannenhoffer states, "I cannot stress enough that a child's experience with food allergies is strongly affected by the behaviors of those around them. Unfortunately, sometimes a child will have experiences with insensitive people and the child will feel some level of feeling different which might generate frustrations. However, if a child is in a socially and emotionally secure environment, then having food allergies is no more significant than having to wear glasses or braces. Interestingly, I have found in my experience that, given the opportunity, food allergies can actually help children bond with each other rather than separate them. I teach that being different is not a negative, but something to be viewed as a positive. We are raising children in a world where they are exposed to special needs and differences every day. They need to be taught tolerance and acceptance."

While the children can be more easily taught and molded, the parents can be more difficult. Ms. Dannenhoffer believes, "Adults have a more difficult time adjusting to things in general. I can imagine that socially, parents of food allergic children might feel different. It may affect the places they go and the social events they can attend. I can only imagine the emotional burden would be overwhelming. Knowing how a parent worries about his or her child's safety normally, I cannot imagine how one must feel having a child with life-threatening allergies. When children are young it may be a little easier knowing you can control almost every aspect of them. But when your child enters school it must be extremely difficult to let go and put your trust in someone else." Throughout childhood there are many decisions to be made and Ms. Dannenhoffer hopes that parents can adjust for their child's food allergies without second guessing their choices.

Some parents whose children don't have food allergies feel that they shouldn't have to be burdened with food allergy rules. Ms. Dannenhoffer has experienced, "There are always parents who just don't get it. They complain that the only thing their child will eat is peanut butter and jelly so they pack peanut butter and crackers in their child's snack or send in cupcakes for his or her birthday. My answer to that is, 'Too bad—we are the adults here so we have to do everything in our power to prevent any and all children from being hurt.' If it were their child, they would feel the same." Ms. Dannenhoffer believes that in general, "The public is very unaware and under-educated about food allergies." People might feel, "I need my hazelnut coffee in the morning." She says, "This is simply ridiculous. In all honesty, I had to make huge adjustments to my diet when I had allergies in my classroom. I'm a peanut butter lover. But I've given it up and am now extremely conscience of where I eat nuts. I think kids are much more flexible and willing to adjust than adults. If you provide fun alternatives to nuts, kids are much more receptive."

Over the past five to ten years, most schools have developed food allergy policies, reports Ms. Dannenhoffer, "The policy can vary from peanut-free schools to peanut-free tables in the cafeteria. Now we have had more peanut-free classrooms as well. Schools have been forced to react to this epidemic. Unfortunately, I have seen a rise in other severe food allergies such as egg and dairy. The focus seems to be on nut allergies though. As little as the general public knows about nut allergies, they are less aware of other food allergies."

More improvements can be made through communication and education. Ms. Dannenhoffer believes, "Every school must have a written policy that is well communicated with all staff and parents. When a teacher is notified that she has a student with food allergies in her room, it should not be a scramble to get things in order. Until you have been through it, you cannot even begin to comprehend the complexity of having food allergies in the classroom. It should be better explained to teachers. It shouldn't be left up to them depending upon whether or not they are conscientious enough to find out what they should do."

Educating all the teachers and other school staff members is imperative. Ms. Dannenhoffer explains, "I think appropriate grade level materials and resources should be made available to all teachers and staff. There are some fantastic free resources online that school principals and parents can order and make available to teachers. While some teachers take it as seriously as they should, not all do. This is sometimes due to a lack of trying, or lack of education, or plainly ignoring it. Some teachers will view it as just protecting themselves legally. Others see it as a moral responsibility."

Parents can help to improve the communication and education of the teachers and school staff. Ms. Dannenhoffer recommends, "Be proactive! Educate the classroom teacher to the best of your ability. Do not assume that he or she has any experience or background with allergies. Do not even assume that your child's allergies have been communicated to the classroom teacher. There can be a lapse of time in the beginning of a school year when teachers have not yet received notice of allergies. It is crucial that teachers be informed with as much notice as possible. This is key in order to educate the parents of other classmates. Provide the teacher with as much information as possible, including a list of foods your child *can't* have. Or if it's easier, provide a list of foods your child *can* have. Be sure to include snack foods on the list so your child can be included in birthdays and classroom celebrations. Together with your child, create a special snack box of things your child can have when the provided snack is in question.

"For example," she continues, "Johnny brings in cupcakes and Mrs. Smith isn't sure...your child can simply pick from his snack box. Be sure the foods in his snack box are special and things that your child enjoys. This can ease a child's feeling different or left out. Ask your child's teacher to discuss the allergy with the whole class, making them aware of its importance. If the allergy requires that your child not have any exposure to a particular food, parents of other students must be notified. In my experience, this happens most often with nut allergies. Remember that in most elementary schools, children eat in the room on a fairly regular basis including a daily snack. My advice to parents is that you give your child's teacher an EpiPen® Jr. and a lesson on how to use it along with written authorization that they can give it if needed. In some states teachers are not authorized to give medication by law. However, in my experience, it will most likely take minutes to notify someone and get a nurse on the scene. Those minutes can mean the difference between life and death. If I had authorization from the parent and an understanding that they wouldn't sue me...I'd do it if it meant saving a child's life." Understanding the teacher's perspective is important. We need to make sure that the parents and teachers work together as a team to protect the safety of the child. Everyone only wants the best for the child.

Communication and education are essential, but it might not be necessary to prepare a detailed 504 Disability Plan. Ms. Dannenhoffer states, "In my experience, a 504 Plan is not necessary with children who have food allergies. 504 Plans are more commonly used when health impairments affect school academic performance. The only reason I would feel that a 504 would be helpful is if it is your only line of defense to communicate your child's allergies to school staff from year to year. Otherwise, it really won't impact your child's educational experience." More importantly, Ms. Dannenhoffer recommends, "Educate yourself as much as possible and educate your child's classroom teachers because they are with your child for a large part of their day and have the ability to change your child's immediate surroundings. They can also adjust the attitudes about allergies in the classroom. Furthermore, Administrators and Boards of Education have the ability to change school wide policies if necessary."

In addition to working with your child's teacher and school, make sure to work with your child. Ms. Dannenhoffer feels, "Parents should be sensitive to children. Tell your child that you love them no matter what. Explain that everyone has differences. Make sure he understands the severity of his circumstances. Don't wait to educate him. If he grows up with the appropriate strategies, he won't know any different. This will simply be the way it is and he will learn to cope. Do not underestimate your child's ability to understand his allergy. Educate him as much as possible. Do not be afraid to explain to him what can happen if he eats the wrong thing. Teach him to ask an adult whether he can eat something. If children (and adults) know that food can be a matter of life and death, they will refrain from eating things they know they shouldn't. This can be very helpful at times when your child is faced with avoiding temptation. Have your child wear a medical alert bracelet. Have it engraved with the specific allergies and foods to avoid. Tell your child how to administer an EpiPen® Jr. if he has one. You cannot be with your child at all times and he is his best ally in those times."

Angela Racine is a middle school teacher and mother of two. She earned a Bachelor of Science in education with a specialty in kindergarten through twelve grades for special education. She taught special education for fifth and sixth grades for seven years then taught multi-age middle school for an additional eight years. She knew she wanted to be a teacher during her own grammar school years. Later, tutoring others through the National Honor Society, including an exceptional Vietnamese student in science, further inspired her to become a teacher.

During Ms. Racine's fifteen years of teaching, she has seen a rise in food allergies. She states, "About four years ago, I noticed that there were more food allergies in all grade levels. The peanut and tree nut allergies were the most common and severe. It seems that over the past four years the incidence of allergies has sort of ebbed and flowed, appearing more significant in some years, then less in others." Ms. Racine points out that her school system has made provisions for peanut allergic students by having peanut-free tables in the cafeteria, but the school still allows peanuts in the school because no student has been so highly allergic to peanuts as to require a complete ban on peanuts. She notes that some neighboring schools have banned peanuts for the entire school. "Schools now make it part of their responsibility to keep all children safe. In the past, safety was not as big an issue—but the level of attention given to safety over the past several years has grown due to the rise in food allergies. For instance, our school doesn't allow peanuts or tree nuts in the classrooms, just the cafeterias," she explains.

Ms. Racine points out, "Teaching middle school children, especially fifth and sixth graders, has its benefits in handling food allergies. Unlike younger children entering kindergarten or other elementary grades, by the time a child is in fifth or sixth grade, he is well aware of his food allergies and what he can and cannot eat. He can monitor himself. It is much more challenging to handle food allergies of children in the lower grades. For this reason, I recommend that a parent always sit down with the teacher prior to the beginning of the school year to discuss the child's food allergy, the symptoms and the treatment. It is imperative that the teacher be educated before a situation arises in the classroom, especially for the youngest children. For that matter, the school nurse and even the principal should be included in the discussions as well."

Ms. Racine continues, "Other provisions that should be made are to educate all the students about food allergies." She explains, "In our school the school nurse gives a presentation in the beginning of the school year. The nurse doesn't point out which child has the food allergy, to avoid making that child uncomfortable, but instead says, 'There is a child in our class who has food allergies.' If the nurse is not well educated on food allergies or willing to give a presentation to the students, then a parent should go into the classroom to do the presentation." For instance, she recalls a situation in which, "A mother of a non-verbal autistic child came to the class at the beginning of the year to speak with the other children about her child. Her purpose in doing this was to try to answer questions about her child *before* the other children experienced any confusion or frustration with her child. She hoped that if the other children were informed with some answers ahead of time, then they would be able to interact with her child more easily. This made the environment better for everyone including her child and even the teacher. It was indeed very helpful."

"For food allergies," Ms. Racine advises, "it is important to have excellent, up front, proactive communication about the child's food allergy. Parents should make appointments to talk to the teachers and nurses before the school year starts. Communication with the other parents can be helpful as well. For instance, one parent sent a flier home to all of the other parents in the class to explain her child's food allergy and to request that they not give certain foods to his or her children when coming to school. All communication is good. Sometimes people worry a little bit about confidentiality, but in this situation the more important thing is communications and sharing information. The more people know the better they will understand and be able to handle the situation. The biggest problem is ignorance. Without firsthand experience, it can be difficult for a parent to understand and accept fully what he is being told with respect to another child's food allergy."

If the parents feel that the school is not providing a safe environment for their child then a 504 Plan can be prepared by the parent and submitted to the school. Ms. Racine believes, "Setting up 504 Plan is a really smart thing to do. It will protect a child's right to an education." For instance, she recalls, "One time a parent was upset that her child could not have peanut butter. It was clear to the teacher that the severity of the allergic child's situation was such that it was necessary to eliminate all peanuts from the environment. In that situation the unwilling parent had to be educated through a discussion. No leeway was given. A 504 Plan can be used to back up the teacher's request to the unwilling parent."

Ms. Racine explains, "Education extends across teachers, staff, parents and students. It is important to have the students understand and be educated about allergies. Our middle school students are taught about how to care for each other and it pays off. One time there was a student who was running in cross-country track practice after school one day. She was stung by a bee. Not knowing that she was allergic, she began to experience anaphylactic symptoms—her lips began to swell. Her friends ran with her back to the school. They did not leave her to run back alone. Once at the school, she was given the appropriate EpiPen® dose and brought to the hospital. Because her friends were educated in allergic reactions, their actions and care may have saved her life. It is so important that the other students are aware of allergies so they can help at these grades."

"If educated in a sensitive way," Ms. Racine states, "I believe the children in middle school are supportive of their peers who have food allergies. I might not hear every single thing that goes on with my fifth and sixth graders, but I hear a lot. Based upon what I hear and watch there isn't teasing of children with food allergies. For instance, we have the peanut-free table in the cafeteria and I have never seen a child sitting alone at that table for lunch. If it were to occur, a teacher would intervene to invite another student to sit with the child who has the allergies, but it really has never been a problem. I have never had a parent call me to complain that the other children are mistreating her child because of her child's food allergy. By the time children are in fifth and sixth grade, they have friends who are supportive and accepting of their food allergies. The parents of the other children are supportive too, by preparing them lunches and snacks that are peanut-free or tree nut-free."

Ms. Racine says, "In addition to the improvements made in schools during the past five years or so, there is always room for more improvements." She continues, "Improvements that can be made include educating the nurse *well* so that she can give informative and well-prepared presentations to the students. Additionally, the presentations should be to the entire school class, not just affected classrooms. Literature could be improved so that teachers have materials to use to teach the students and parents. The literature should include a story that can effectively show the students how it can feel to suffer a food allergy." For instance, Ms. Racine explained how her own son recently was taught how it felt to suffer an asthma attack. Each student was given a straw to breathe through. He soon felt the labored and shortness of breath caused by not getting enough air. It was very effective to demonstrate the feeling to him and others. Furthermore, having a full-time nurse, instead of a part-time nurse is important because anaphylactic shock can occur any time during the day. Ms. Racine recommends, "In addition to proactive communication with the teacher, nurse and other school staff, it is important to develop relationships with other parents of children who have food allergies. Form a team to help educate others to build safe guards and care for all allergic children."

CHAPTER 51: TRAVEL

One day when our first son was about one year of age, I was food shopping at the local grocery store. There was an older gentleman who came up to my son and me. He began to talk to us and told me how adorable my son was. He reached out and took his hand in such a loving way and my son held onto his finger tightly. Normally, I didn't like it when people touched my son's hands because he would then put them into his mouth, but this time I didn't really mind, much to my own surprise. The gentleman said, "You have to share your baby with people like me." My curiosity peaked and I gathered the courage to ask, "Why?" Then the gentleman began to tell me that he once had two daughters. He told me that he and his wife traveled a lot when his daughters were young. Then, in one country, one of his daughters caught Meningitis and died, and then several years later, the other daughter died of another horrible disease contracted far from home. My heart went out to this man. It seemed so unfair that he lost both of his children. He was truly a kind spirit.

My reason for telling this story is to remind you that the environment is different when you are traveling away from your home. When away, you will encounter things that your body is not used to encountering and it can be dangerous, perhaps especially with a food-allergic child whose immune system is already over-stressed. Getting vaccinations prior to traveling, learning the local emergency telephone numbers from cell or land line phones and confirming airline guidelines for food and EpiPen® Jr. administration are essential, especially when traveling with a child who has food allergies. The following airline guidelines and telephone numbers may become out of date after the printing of this book. Please check to confirm them prior to traveling.

Airline Guidelines

According to an article entitled, "What Can You Bring on the Airplane? No Liquids Allowed Onboard,"[158] the Transportation Security Administration (TSA) defines what can be brought on the plane for international flights:

- Any food purchased in the international departures lounge must be consumed before boarding.

- Prescription medicines and medical items sufficient and essential for the flight, such as a diabetic kit, except in liquid form unless verified as authentic. You will need a prescription to carry on medicines.

- For those traveling with an infant: Baby food, milk (the contents of each bottle must be tasted by the accompanying passenger), and sanitary items sufficient and essential for the flight, such as diapers, wipes, creams, and diaper disposal bags.

According to article entitled, "Travel with Kids,"[159] the TSA has a 3-1-1 for carry-on motto:

- Toiletries (and other liquids, gels, lotions, etc.) must each be in a three ounce container (or smaller);

- Pack these items together in a one quart sized, clear, plastic, zip-top bag;

- One such bag per passenger is allowed, and must be removed from your carry-on bag and placed in a bin to go through the screening machine.

And additional food related rules include:

- You can bring bottled water IF you first pass through the security gate, and then buy the water (or other beverage) in the secure boarding area.

- Food items such as jams, salsas, sauces, syrups and dips will not be allowed through the checkpoint unless they are in containers three ounces or less and in the passenger's one quart zip-top bag.

- Exceptions: Formula, breast milk, baby food. Parents of babies, of course, have to bring aboard nourishment for their little ones. Baby formula and milk are allowed in quantities greater than three ounces and don't need to be packed in the zip-top bag. Keep in mind that you must be traveling with a baby or toddler and take only amounts needed for the plane trip (pack the rest in your checked luggage). You'll need to declare these items for inspection at the security checkpoint.

- Parents can also stock their carry-on bag with baby food in cans or jars and gel or liquid-filled teethers for babies.

Also check the Transportation Security Administration's web site for travel carry on rules prior to your travel as the rules may change between this writing and your travel date. The TSA's web site is located at: http://www.tsa.gov/travelers/index.shtm.

According to an article entitled, "Airline Allergy Policies,"[160] by Victoria Groce, the airlines have the following guidelines and policies.

American Airlines: Peanut Allergy: American recognizes that some passengers are allergic to peanuts. Although we do not serve peanuts, we do serve other nut products and there may be trace elements of unspecified peanut ingredients, including peanut oils, in meal and snacks. We make no provisions to be peanut-free. Additionally, other customers may bring peanuts on board. Therefore, we cannot guarantee customers will not be exposed to peanuts during flight and strongly encourage customers to take all necessary medical precautions to prepare for the possibility of exposure. American Airlines offers special meals to meet specific dietary needs at your request on select flights. Specifications for all medical-needs diets are approved and monitored by a Registered Dietitian. Nutritional requirements are based on the whole meal rather than individual components.

Continental: Vegan (strict) vegetarian meals are available for those customers who exclude all foods derived from animals (including meat, poultry, fish, shellfish, honey, eggs, and dairy products) or their by-products from their diets. Gluten-free meals are available for those customers who need to limit their intake of gluten (or gliadin, a protein fraction of gluten) a substance found in wheat, barley, rye and oats.

Delta: When you notify us that you have a peanut allergy, we'll create a buffer zone of three rows in front of and three rows behind your seat. We'll also advise cabin service to board extra pretzels, which will allow our flight attendants to serve only pretzels within this area. Gate agents will be notified in case you'd like to pre-board and cleanse the immediate seating area. We'll do everything we can, but unfortunately we still can't guarantee that the flight will be completely peanut-free.

Northwest Airlines: Northwest recognizes that some customers are allergic to peanuts or tree nuts (almonds, cashews, etc.), and that exposure to peanuts or tree nuts can result in dire, even fatal, consequences for customers with the most severe allergies. Northwest Airlines cannot guarantee an environment free of any allergens, including peanuts, peanut dust, peanut oil, or peanut remnants. Northwest does not serve peanuts or products made with or containing peanuts. Northwest does, however, serve products containing tree nuts. The tree nuts and other products served onboard, including meals, snack boxes and snack mixes, may be processed or packaged in factories that produce peanut or other nut products. Peanuts, products made from peanut oil, and other nuts may be brought onboard by any passenger. Northwest does not remove tree nut products from aircraft or perform any special cleaning to remove peanut or tree nut residue. Northwest does, at the request of a customer with a peanut allergy, make an announcement in the gate area and onboard the flight requesting that passengers please refrain from eating peanut products during that flight. We suggest the following precautions for customers with peanut/tree nut allergies when flying on Northwest:

- Upon arriving at the airport, advise the gate agent working your flight (including connecting flights) so the agent may make the necessary announcement in the gate area prior to boarding;

- Consider taking the aircraft's first flight of the day whenever possible, as aircraft receive a more thorough cleaning overnight than they do during the day; and

- Consider the possibility of exposure, particularly when accepting any in-flight snack or meal. They are encouraged to bring their own food with them. Customers may wear face masks or use respirators (note: there are special procedures for respirators, including advance notice).

Southwest Airlines: Southwest Airlines is unable to guarantee a peanut-free or allergen-free flight. We have procedures in place to assist our customers with severe allergies to peanut dust and will make every attempt not to serve packaged peanuts on the aircraft when our customers alert us to their allergy to peanut dust. If the reservation is made online, there is a field to indicate a peanut allergy. We suggest that customers with an allergy to peanut dust:

- Book their travel on early morning flights, as our aircraft undergo a thorough cleaning only at the end of the day;

- Check in at the departure gate one hour prior to departure and notify our customer service agent at the gate of the allergy to complete a Peanut Dust Allergy form;

- Inform our flight attendant upon boarding. Flight attendants will make every effort to serve an alternate snack, but some of snacks may contain peanut particles, peanut oil, or have been packaged in a peanut facility;

- Read the ingredients on any packaged snack before consumption. Of course, all customers are welcome to bring their own snacks with them.

Although following the above procedures will ensure peanuts are not served on a flight, Southwest cannot prevent other customers from bringing peanuts or products containing peanuts onboard our flights. In addition, Southwest cannot give assurances that remnants of peanuts and/or peanut dust/oil will not remain on the aircraft floor, seats, or tray tables from flights earlier in the aircraft's routing.

U.S. Airways: Peanut Allergies: U.S. Airways recognizes that some of our passengers are allergic to peanut products. However, due to last-minute aircraft changes and the possibility that other passengers may bring peanuts onboard, we cannot guarantee that no peanut products will be onboard. Because we cannot accommodate "peanut-free" snack requests and the possibility that peanut-related ingredients may be contained in meals, we encourage passengers to bring their own food items onboard the flight.

Special Meals: Special meals are only available on transatlantic flights in envoy and main cabin. Special meals must be ordered at least twenty-four hours in advance and include: Asian begetarian, baby, bland, children's, diabetic, gluten-free, Hindu, Kosher, lacto ovo (no meat, but dairy and egg), low calorie, low fat/low cholesterol, low sodium, Moslem, non-lactose, peanut-free, and vegan.

United Airlines: Below are the guidelines United follows in preparing gluten-free meals for customers diagnosed with celiac disease. Prohibited: Wheat and wheat flour, barley, oats and rye, sauces, breads, cakes, biscuits, pastry, sausages/sausage meats, pasta, gravy mixes/stock cubes. Allowed: Meat/poultry, fresh fish, rice, fresh fruits, vegetables, corn, salt, pepper, herbs, spices, potatoes, eggs, aged cheese, dairy products, sugars, preserves, margarine, tapioca, vegetable oils, yogurt, dried beans, peas and chocolate.

Not all airlines have written policies. The following airlines have no written allergy policy as of May 2007:

- AirTran Airways
- Continental Airlines, except as stated above.
- JetBlue
- Airlines, except as stated above.

International Emergency Telephone Numbers

If you are planning a trip, you should check the laws and typical language used to discuss anaphylaxis and its treatment. Check emergency procedures for the method of transportation you will be taking. Ask your child's doctor to learn if you should or can have a doctor's note to bring the EpiPen® Jr. or any other medication with you.

- Confirm that you can bring your EpiPen® Jr. on the plane, train, bus or subway.

- Confirm that you can bring your EpiPen® Jr. into the destination country.

- Confirm food guidelines and allergy policies for the airline(s) you are flying.

- Confirm that EpiPen® Jrs. are allowed to be administered by ambulatory staff. For instance:

    - In Australia, when calling an ambulance, you must specify that an *"intensive care for a child"* ambulance must be requested else there will not be an EpiPen® Jr. on board or a person qualified to administer it;

    - In Italy, when an ambulance is called you must specify *"anaphylaxis"*;

    - In New Zealand, you must specify, "Someone is having an anaphylactic reaction and *adrenaline/epinephrine* is needed." Not all ambulances carry epinephrine, and only paramedics are authorized to administer it;

- In the United Kingdom, you must say, "The patient is suffering from anaphylaxis and needs *adrenaline*," as this is the common term in the U.K. for epinephrine; and

- In parts of *rural* New Zealand ambulance officers are often volunteer first-aid personnel and don't have paramedic qualifications, *so can't administer an adrenaline.*

You should also verify emergency numbers for each country to which you travel and through which you travel. The following information was obtained from the Santa Clara Fire Department.[161] For "local numbers only" check with the destination airport staff and hotel staff for local emergency telephone numbers and recheck the information if you travel to various locations at your destination. Confirm the emergency phone number listed below has not changed, just before the time of your trip.

Afghanistan: local numbers only
Albania: 17
Algeria: 21606666
American Samoa: 911
Andorra: 118
Angola: local numbers only
Anguilla: 911
Antarctica (McMurdo Station): 911
Antigua & Barbuda: 999 / 911
Argentina: 101
Armenia: 103
Aruba: 911
Ascension Island: 6000
Australia: 000 (112 on cell phone)
Austria: 112 / 122
Azerbaijan (Baku): 3
Azores: 112
Bahamas: 911

Bahrain: 999
Bali: 112
Bangladesh (Dhaka): 199
Barbados: 115 / 119
Belgium: 112 (cell) / 101
Belarus: 3
Belize: 911
Benin: local numbers only
Bermuda: 911
Bhutan: local numbers only
Bolivia (Lapaz): 118
Bonaire: 14 or 5997 8004
Bornio (Sabah): 999
Bosnia-Herzegovina: 124
Botswana: 997 / 911
Brazil: 911
Bosnia: 94
British Virgin Islands: 999
Brunei: 991
Bulgaria: 150
Burkina Faso: local numbers only
Burma/Myanmar: 999
Burundi: local numbers only
Cambodia, The Kingdom of (Phnom Penh): 119
Cameroon: local numbers only
Canada (AB, MB, NB, NS, ON, PE, QU): 911
Canada (BC, NF, SK): 911 local only[1]
Canada (NT):
Canada (NU): local only
Canada (YK): 3 dig+3333
Canary Islands: 112
Cape Verde: 131
Cayman Islands: 911
Central African Republic: local numbers only
Chad: local numbers only
Chile: 131
China, The People's Republic of: 999 / 120 (Beijing)
Colombia: 119
Comoros Islands: local numbers only
Congo: local numbers only

Cook Islands: 998
Costa Rica: 911
Côte d'Ivoire: local numbers only
Croatia: 112
Cuba: 26811
Curaçao: 112
Cyprus: 112
Czech Republic: 112/155
Congo, Democratic Republic of Zaïre: local numbers only
Denmark: 112
Djibouti: local numbers only
Dominica, Commonwealth of: 999
Dominican Republic: 911
East Timor: 112
Ecuador: 131
Egypt: 0
El Salvador: 911
England: 112 / 999
Equatorial Guinea: local numbers only
Eritrea: local numbers only
Estonia: 112
Ethiopia: local numbers only
Faeroe Islands (Denmark): 112
Falkland Islands: 999
Fiji: 000 / 911
Finland: 112
France: 112 / 15
French Guiana: 112 / 15
Gabon: local numbers only
Gaborone: 997 / 911
Gambia, The: 16
Georgia: 3
Germany: 112
Ghana: local numbers only
Gibraltar: 999
Greece: 112 / 166
Greenland: local numbers only
Grenada: 434
Guadeloupe: 18
Guam: 911

Guatamala: 123
Guernsey: 999
Guinea Bissau: local numbers only
Guinea Republic: local numbers only
Guyana: 999
Haiti: 118
Honduras: 195^2 / 37 8654
Hong Kong: 999
Hungary: 112
Iceland: 112
India: 102
Indonesia: 118
Iran: 115
Iraq: local numbers only
Ireland, Republic of: 112 / 999
Israel: 101
Italy: 118
Jamaica: 110
Japan: 119
Jersey: 999
Jordan: 193
Kazakhstan: 3
Kenya: 999
Kiribati: 994
Kosovo: 94
Korea: local numbers only
Korea: The Republic of (South Korea): 119
Kuwait: 777
Kyrgyzstan: 103
Laos: local numbers only
Latvia: 03 / 112
Lebanon: 1401
Lesotho: 121
Liberia: 911 (cell phones only)
Libya: 119
Liechtenstein: 112
Lithuania: 112
Luxembourg: 112 / 113
Macau: 999
Macedonia: 94

Madagascar: local numbers only
Madeira: 112
Malawi: 998
Malaysia: 999
Maldives Republic: 102
Mali: 15
Malta: 112
Marianas Island: 911
Martinique: 18
Mauritius: 114
Mayotte: 15
Menorca: 112
México: 65
Micronesia, Federated States of: local numbers only
Moldavia: 903
Monaco: 112
Mongolia: 103
Montserrat: 911
Morocco: 15
Moyotte: 15
Mozambique: 117
Namibia: 2032276
Nauru: local numbers only
Nepal: 2280941
Netherlands (Holland): 112
Netherlands Antilles: 912
New Caledonia: 18
New Zealand: 111
Nicaragua: 265 1761
Niger: local numbers only
Nigeria: 199
Niue: 998
Northern Ireland: 112 / 999
Norway: 112 / 110
Oman: 999
Pakistan: 115
Palau: 911
Palestine: 101
Panama[3]: 269-9778
Paraguay: 0

Peru: 011 / 5114
Philippines: 166 / 117
Pitcairn Islands: no telephone system
Poland: 112 / 999
Portugal: 112 (115 for forest fires)
Puerto Rico: 911
Qatar: 999 / 118
Réunion: 15 / 112
Romania: 961 / 962
Russia: 112
Russian Federation: 3
Rwanda: local numbers only
Saba: 912
Sabah (Borneo): 999
Samoa: 999
San Marino: 113
São Tomé and Principe: local numbers only
Sarawak: 994
Saudi Arabia: 997
Scotland: 112 / 999
Scilly, Isles of: 999
Senegal: local numbers only
Seychelles: 999
Sierra Leone: 999
Singapore: 995
Slovak Republic (Slovakia): 155
Slovenia: 112
Solomon Islands: 911
Somalia: local numbers only
South Africa: 10177
South Africa (Cape Town): 107
S. Georgia Is./S. Sandwich Is.: no telephone system
Srpska, Republic of: 94
Spain: 112
Sri Lanka: 1 691095 / 699935
St Eustatius: 140
St Eustatius: 911
St Helena: 911
St Kitts & Nevis: 911
St Lucia: 999 / 911

St Maarten: 911 / 542-2111
St Vincent & the Grenadines: 999 / 911
Sudan: local numbers only
Suriname: local numbers only
Swaziland: local numbers only
Sweden: 112
Switzerland: 144
Syrian Arab Republic (Syria): 110
Tahiti - French Polynesia: 15
Taiwan (Republic of China): 119
Tajikistan: 3
Tanzania: 112 / 999
Thailand: 191
Tibet: unknown
Tonga: 911
Trinidad & Tobago: 990
Tunisia: 190
Turkey: 112
Turkmenistan: 3
Turks and Caicos Islands: 999 / 911
Tuvalu / Ellice Is.: 911
Uganda: 112 (mobile) / 999 (fixed)
Ukraine: 03 / 118
United Arab Emirates (Abu Dhabi): 998 / 999
United Kingdom: 112 / 999
United States: 911
Uruguay: 999 / 911
US Virgin Islands: 911
Uzbekistan: 3
Vanuatu: 22 100
Vatican City: 113
Venezuela: 171
Vietnam: 115
Wake Island: no telephone system
Western Sahara: 150
Western Samoa: 999
Yemen, Republic of: local numbers only
Yugoslavia (Serbia & Montenegro): 94
Zambia: 999
Zimbabwe: 994 / 999

CONCLUSION

The purpose of this book is to provide social, emotional and practical guidance in parenting your young food allergic child. Knowing that others have successfully dealt with food allergies should give you some confidence and reading their stories will likely have given you some ideas for dealing with food allergies. However the different perspectives of doctors demonstrate that more research is needed for more conclusive information on testing, treating and possibly curing food allergies.

Let's come together and ask our government to give more attention to the research of food allergies. The current trend indicates that food allergies are affecting more children every day. If enough requests are heard by our government and related organizations, perhaps more funding will be allocated to perform the much-needed studies. In 2005 about $7 million was allocated. In 2008, the director of NIAID is hoping for $13 million. But researchers state that $50 million is needed to properly address the situation.

You can help by asking our government to conduct studies. Your specific interest might be:

- What research can be done to better diagnose and treat food allergies in young children?

- How do food allergies affect autism?

- How do food allergies affect ADHD?

- How do food allergies affect asthma?

- How do genetically modified foods affect food allergies?

- How to pesticides affect food allergies?

- How do hormones and antibiotics in our livestock affect food allergies?

- Why don't labeling laws require all ingredients in artificial colors/flavors and natural colors/flavors to be listed?

There are several organizations leading the quest of researching food allergies and helping those with them. For instance, the Asthma and Allergy Foundation of America (AAFA) is the oldest and largest allergy patient advocacy organization in the world. Founded in 1953, AAFA's mission is to provide practical information, community based services and support through a national network of chapters and support groups. AAFA develops food allergy educational programs and materials, organizes state and national advocacy efforts, and funds research to find better treatments and cures. (1233 20th Street, NW, Suite 402, Washington, DC, 20036 USA, www.aafa.org, info@aafa.org, 1-800-7-ASTHMA).

In addition to FAAN and AAFA, the American Academy of Allergy Asthma and Immunology (AAAAAI) and Food Allergy Initiative (FAI) support similar goals. Please see the References section below for all of these organizations' missions and contact information.

To participate in asking our government for more funding, research and support you can write a letter. Feel free to use the guidelines on FAAN's web site at: http://www.foodallergy.org/advocacy/index.html or photocopy and fill in information in the sample letter on the following page to ask your congressman to support increased funding for food allergy research. *Locate your senators' or representatives' addresses by calling the U.S. House and Senate switchboard at (202) 224-3121 or check www.house.gov and www.senate.gov.*

Good luck and remember that you are not alone and we must all stand together to request more funding for research and answers.

_____,_____200_

The Honorable _____

I am writing to express my support for:

    1) The passage of the Food Allergy and Anaphylaxis Management Act (S.1232 in the Senate, HR.2063 in the House). I understand this bill passed in the House of Representatives on April 8, 2008, but remains to be passed by the Senate.

    Its purpose is to, "Require the Secretary of Health and Human Services to develop and make available to local educational agencies a policy to manage the risk of food allergy and anaphylaxis in schools to be implemented on a voluntary basis only. Direct that such policy address: (1) a parental obligation to provide the school with information regarding a student's food allergy and risk of anaphylaxis; (2) creation of an individual health care plan tailored to each student with a documented risk for anaphylaxis; (3) communication strategies between schools and emergency medical services; (4) strategies to reduce the risk of exposure in classrooms and common areas; (5) food allergy management training of school personnel; and (6) authorization and training of school personnel to administer epinephrine when the school nurse is not immediately available. It allows the Secretary to award grants to assist local educational agencies in implementing such food allergy management guidelines."[162]

    2) Increase federal funding for food allergy research from the current requested amount of about $13M to $50M, as recommended by the researchers who gathered at Children's Memorial. Dr. Robert Schleimer, chief of the Allergy-Immunology Division at Northwestern University Feinberg School of Medicine stated, "There are enough children with food allergies to do the thorough research needed to determine not only how many are now affected, but also to find better treatment."[163]

Thank you for considering these requests.

Sincerely,

_____

References

National Institute of Allergy and Infectious Diseases (NIAID). The National Institute of Allergy and Infectious Diseases (NIAID), part of the National Institutes of Health (NIH), is the nation's principal supporter of food allergy research. NIAID's broad support of basic research in allergy and immunology provides an increasingly better understanding of the immune system and how, in certain people, foods trigger an allergic reaction. NIAID supports clinical trials that are attempting to alter the body's immune system so that it no longer triggers allergic reactions. NIAID also supports research on basic immunology, transplantation and immune-related disorders, including autoimmune diseases, asthma and allergies.

31 Center Drive MSC 2520
Bethesda, MD 20892
www3.niaid.nih.gov/
niaidnews@niaid.nih.gov
301-496-5717

Asthma and Allergy Foundation of America (AAFA). The Asthma and Allergy Foundation of America (AAFA) is the oldest and largest allergy patient advocacy organization in the world. Founded in 1953, AAFA's mission is to provide practical information, community based services and support through a national network of chapters and support groups. AAFA develops food allergy educational programs and materials, organizes state and national advocacy efforts, and funds research to find better treatments and cures.

1233 20th Street, NW, Suite 402
Washington, DC, 20036 USA
www.aafa.org
info@aafa.org
1-800-7-ASTHMA

American Academy of Allergy Asthma and Immunology (AAAAAI). Established in 1943, the AAAAI works to support our 6,500 members worldwide in providing high quality, compassionate health care for those with allergy, asthma and immunologic disorders by: Providing advocacy and support for patients and the allergy/immunology specialists who provide their care; providing education and information about allergy/immunology for its members, other healthcare professionals, patients and the public; fostering and disseminating research and new information in allergy/immunology; and enhancing and supporting academic allergy/immunology programs

555 East Wells Street, Suite 1100
Milwaukee, WI 53202-3823
www.aaaai.org
info@aaaai.org
1-414-272-6071

Food Allergy and Anaphylaxis Network (FAAN). The Food Allergy & Anaphylaxis Network (FAAN) was established in 1991. FAAN's membership now stands at close to 30,000 worldwide and includes families, dietitians, nurses, physicians, school staff, and representatives from government agencies and the food and pharmaceutical industries. FAAN serves as the communication link between the patient and others.

11781 Lee Jackson Hwy., Suite 160
Fairfax, VA 22033-3309
www.foodallergy.org/about.html
faan@foodallergy.org
1-800-929-4040

Food Allergy Initiative (FAI). The Food Allergy Initiative (FAI) is a 501(c)(3) non-profit organization that raises funds toward the effective treatment and cure for food allergies. Funds raised by FAI are invested in research that seeks to find a cure and improve clinical treatment. FAI has established a Medical Advisory Board to identify and recommend the most promising research in the United States and around the world. FAI also provides grants to entities that serve and support food allergic patients and their families at the Mount Sinai School of Medicine in New York City. In addition, it is FAI's mission to raise public awareness about the seriousness of food allergies. Through effective educational programs and public information, FAI heightens awareness of food allergies and the danger of anaphylaxis among the media, health care workers, education and child care professionals, while also working with the nation's policy makers to create a safer environment and improve care for the food allergic population.

1414 Avenue of the Americas, Suite 1804
New York, NY 10019
www.foodallergyinitiative.org
info@foodallergyinitiative.org
1-212-207-1974

American Academy of Pediatrics (AAP). The American Academy of Pediatrics is an organization of 60,000 pediatricians committed to the attainment of optimal physical, mental, and social health and well-being for all infants, children, adolescents, and young adults.

141 Northwest Point Boulevard
Elk Grove Village, IL 60007-1098
www.aap.org
For specific questions, ask your pediatrician.
If you need a pediatrician see: http://www.aap.org/referral/
1-847-434-4000

END NOTES

[1] "Peanut Allergy," AllergicChild.com, 11/5/07,
<http://www.allergicchild.com/peanut_allergy.htm>, (11/7/07).

[2] "Food Allergy Basics," Food Allergy and Anaphylaxis Network,
<http://www.foodallergy.org/downloads/FABasics.pdf>, (11/7/07).

[3] "Food Allergy & Anaphylaxis Network - Docket No. 2004N-051 6 (2005
FSS)- Pu@ c Comment,"
<http://www.fda.gov/ohrms/DOCKETS/dockets/04n0516/04n-0516-
c000001-01-vol1.pdf>, (11/7/07).

[4] "Allergy Facts and Figures," Asthma and Allergy Foundation of America,
<http://www.aafa.org/display.cfm?id=9&sub=30>, (11/7/07).

[5] "Asthma and Allergic Diseases," National Institute of Allergy and Infectious
Diseases,
<http://www3.niaid.nih.gov/about/overview/profile/fy2003/pdf/SSAR_
ASTHMA.pdf>, (11/ 7/07).

[6] "Allergy Testing for Children," Asthma and Allergy Foundation of America,
<http://www.aafa.org/display.cfm?id=9&sub=20&cont=278>,
(11/7/07).

[7] Dioun, Anahita F., Harris, Sion Kim, Hibberd, Patricia L. (2003) "Is maternal age at delivery related to childhood food allergy?", Pediatric Allergy and Immunology 14 (4), 307–311, doi:10.1034/j.1399-
3038.2003.00063.x, Blackwell Synergy, <http://www.blackwell-
synergy.com/doi/abs/10.1034/j.1399-
3038.2003.00063.x?journalCode=pai> , (11/7/07).

[8] "Food Allergen Labeling and Consumer Protection Act of 2004," U.S. Food
and Drug Administration, August 2, 2004,
<http://www.cfsan.fda.gov/~dms/alrgact.html>, (11/7/2007).

[9] "Food Allergen Labeling and Consumer Protection Act of 2004," U.S. Food
and Drug Administration, August 2, 2004,
<http://www.cfsan.fda.gov/~dms/alrgact.html>, (11/7/2007).

[10] "How do artificial flavors work?" howstuffworks, <http://science.howstuffworks.com/question391.htm>, (11/7/07).

[11] Department of Health and Human Services, "Testimony Subcommittee on Children and Families Committee on Health, Education, Labor, and Pensions United States Senate," May 14, 2008, <http://www3.niaid.nih.gov/about/directors/pdf/foodAllergyHearingStatement.pdf>, (5/19/2008).

[12] Sheehan, Charles, "Scientists see spike in kids' food allergies," Chicago Tribune, 9 June 2006, <http://www.non-gm-farmers.com/news_details.asp?ID=2789>, (12/31/2007).

[13] Bucchini, Luca Ph.D., and Goldman, Lynn R., M.D. MPH, "A Snapshot of Federal Research on Food Allergy," A report commissioned by the Pew Initiative on Food and Biotechnology, June 2002, <http://www.pewtrusts.org/uploadedFiles/wwwpewtrustsorg/Reports/Food_and_Biotechnology/hhs_biotech_snapshot.pdf>, (11/7/07).

[14] Vieths, Stefan, "IgE-Mediated food allergy diagnosis: Current status and new perspectives," Journal of Molecular Nutrition & Food Research Volume 51, Issue 1, Pages 135-147, 12/29/2006 <http://www3.interscience.wiley.com/cgi-bin/abstract/114032672/ABSTRACT>, (11/7/07).

[15] "Irritable bowel syndrome", <http://en.wikipedia.org/wiki/Irritable_bowel_syndrome>, (12/18/2007).

[16] Adapted or Reprinted with permission from 'Food Allergies: Just the FactsMyths 1-9, September 2000, Sicherer, S.H., M.D. and familydoctor.org editorial staff, "Manifestations of Food Allergy: Evaluation and Management," American Family Physician, American Academy of Family Physicians, January 15, 1999, <http://familydoctor.org/online/famdocen/home/common/allergies/basics/340.html>, (11/7/07).

[17] "Food Allergy Myths and Realities," International Food Information Council, December 1997, http://www.ific.org/foodinsight/1997/nd/allergyfi697.cfm, (3/24/2008).

[18] Anitei, Stefan, "Food Allergy Myths Busted in the Case of Babies," Softpedia, January 8, 2008, <http://news.softpedia.com/news/Allergy-Food-Myths-Busted-in-the-Case-of-Babies-75555.shtml>, (3/24/2008).

[19] Bateson-Koch, N.D., Carolee, "Five Myths About Food Allergies," Alive, May 2002, <http://www.alive.com/923a3a2.php?subject_bread_cramb=227>, (3/24/2008).

[20] Parentingscience.com, "The dark side of preschool: Peers, social skills, and stress," <http://www.parentingscience.com/preschool-stress.html>, (11/15/07).

[21] Kane, Anthony, "ADHD and Food Allergies. Food allergy symptoms," <http://allergy.usgab.com/post_1177575429.html>, (11/7/07) citing source <www.addadhdadvances.com/>.

[22] Barnes, Henry, "Waldorf Education K-12", October 1991, <http://www.awsna.org/education-k12.html>, (11/7/07).

[23] Pusztai, Arpad, "Genetically Modified Foods: Are They a Risk to Human/Animal Health?", American Institute of Biological Sciences, June 2001, <http://www.actionbioscience.org/biotech/pusztai.html>, (11/7/07).

[24] Human Genome Project Information, "What are Genetically Modified (GM) Foods?" July 24, 2007, <http://www.ornl.gov/sci/techresources/Human_Genome/elsi/gmfood.shtml>, (11/7/07).

[25] Human Genome Project Information, "What are Genetically Modified (GM) Foods?" July 24, 2007, <http://www.ornl.gov/sci/techresources/Human_Genome/elsi/gmfood.shtml>, (11/7/07).

[26] Human Genome Project Information, "What are Genetically Modified (GM) Foods?" July 24, 2007, <http://www.ornl.gov/sci/techresources/Human_Genome/elsi/gmfood.shtml>, (11/7/07).

[27] Leamy, Elisabeth, "Secrets in Your Food – Genetically Modified Food: Is It Safe?" August 21, 2006, ABC News, <http://abcnews.go.com/GMA/Story?id=2337731&page=1>, (11/7/07).

[28] Leamy, Elisabeth, "Secrets in Your Food – Genetically Modified Food: Is It Safe?," August 21, 2006, ABC News, <http://abcnews.go.com/GMA/Story?id=2337731&page=1>, (11/7/07).

[29] The Campaign, "Do you know what is in your food? Is it genetically engineered?", <http://www.thecampaign.org/>, (11/7/07).

[30] Smith, Jeffrey M., "Genetically Engineered Foods May Cause Rising Food Allergies," <http://www.nwrage.org/index.php?name=News&file=article&sid=1789>, (11/7/07).

[31] The Pew Initiative on Food and Biotechnology, "Unlikely Reactions: Identifying Allergies to GM Foods," <http://pewagbiotech.org/buzz/display.php3?StoryID=12>, (11/7/07).

[32] Smith, Jeffrey M., "Genetically Engineered Foods May Cause Rising Food Allergies," <http://www.nwrage.org/index.php?name=News&file=article&sid=1789>, (11/7/07).

[33] Schierow, Linda-Jo, Specialist in Environmental Policy, "Pesticide Residue Regulation: Analysis of Food Quality Protection Act Implementation," November 4, 2002, <http://www.ncseonline.org/nle/crsreports/02Dec/RS20043.pdf>, (11/7/07).

[34] Motala, Dr. Cassiem, Allergy Society of South Africa, "Food Allergy," <http://www.allergysa.org/food.htm>, (11/7/07).

[35] Sumei Liu, Hong-Zhen Hu, Na Gao, Go-Du Wang, Xiyu Wang, Owen C. Peck, Gordon Kim, Yun Xia, and Jackie D. Wood, "Neuroimmune Interactions in Guinea-Pig Stomach and Small Intestine: A Signaling Role for Histamine, Prostaglandins and Leukotrienes," American Physiological Society, submitted June 21, 2002, accepted September 6, 2002,

<http://ajpgi.physiology.org/cgi/content/short/00241.2002v1>, (11/8/07).

36 Woods, J.D., "Histamine, mast cells, and the enteric nervous system in the irritable bowel syndrome, enteritis, and food allergies," 2006 BMJ Publishing Group Ltd & British Society of Gastroenterology, <http://gut.bmj.com/cgi/content/extract/55/4/445>, (11/8/07).

37 Schierow, Linda-Jo, Specialist in Environmental Policy, "Pesticide Residue Regulation: Analysis of Food Quality Protection Act Implementation," November 4, 2002, <http://www.ncseonline.org/nle/crsreports/02Dec/RS20043.pdf>, (11/7/07).

38 Clinical and Experimental Allergy, Volume 37, pages 661-670, 2006, "Farm Milk Linked with Lower Rate of Asthma and Allergies," <http://www.eatwild.com/news.html>, (11/8/07).

39 Cummins, Ronnie, "Frankenfoods, Antibiotics, & Mad Cow: America's Food Safety Crisis Intensifies," 2/1/2001, <http://www.inmotionmagazine.com/geff10.html>, (11/8/07).

40 Kinship Circle, "Dairy & Veal Factories: Human Health," <http://www.kinshipcircle.org/fact_sheets/FactsAboutDairyVealIndu str.pdf>, (11/8/07).

41 Boon, Rosemary, "Food Allergies, Coeliac Disease, Milk Intolerance & Nutritional Issues," <http://home.iprimus.com.au/rboon/FOODALLERGIES.htm>, (11/8/07).

42 Boon, Rosemary, "Food Allergies, Coeliac Disease, Milk Intolerance & Nutritional Issues," <http://home.iprimus.com.au/rboon/FOODALLERGIES.htm>, (11/8/07).

43 Cady, Louis, M.D., "Food Allergy Testing for ADHD and Autism," 3/23/05, <http://www.betterhealthusa.com/public/336.cfm>, (11/9/07).

[44] Alpha Nutrition a division of Environmed Research Inc., Sechelt, British Columbia, Canada, "Food Allergy and Lung Disease," <http://www.nutramed.com/asthma/foodallergy.htm>, (11/9/07).

[45] Yazbak, F. Edward, M.D., F.A.A.P., Journal of American Physicians and Surgeons Volume 8 Number 4 Winter 2003, "Autism in the United States: a Perspective," <http://www.autismtoday.com/articles/Autism-in-the-United-States.htm>, (11/9/07).

[46] Potter, Ned, "CDC Says 300,000 Children Have Autism," May 2, 2006, AB-CNews, <http://www.abcnews.go.com/Health/story?id=1925018&page=1>, (11/9/07).

[47] Yazbak, F. Edward, M.D., F.A.A.P., Journal of American Physicians and Surgeons Volume 8 Number 4 Winter 2003, "Autism in the United States: a Perspective," <http://www.autismtoday.com/articles/Autism-in-the-United-States.htm>, (11/9/07).

[48] Fighting Autism, Thoughtful House Center for Children, <http://www.fightingautism.org/idea/autism.php>, (11/9/07).

[49] Anderson, Anne, "Improve an Autistic Child's Life: Understanding the role of dietary allergens," San Diego Family Magazine, August, 2007.

[50] "Dysfuctional Metabolism, Gastrointestinal and Autoimmune Issues," 2/14/2006, <http://www.mentalhelp.net/poc/view_doc.php?type=doc&id=8773&cn=20>, (11/9/07).

[51] Seroussi, Karyn, "We Cured Our Son's Autism," <http://www.autisminfo.com/seroussi.htm>, (11/9/07).

[52] Lewey, Dr. Scot, "Autism linked to cow's milk protein when GI symptoms present: More thoughts on the brain gut connection," January 3, 2007, <http://thefooddoc.blogspot.com/search?q=Casomorphin+is+protein+fragment+>, (11/9/07).

[53] Bren, Linda, "Food labels identify allergens more clearly," FDA Consumer, 3/1/2006, <http://www.encyclopedia.com/doc/1G1-151662080.html>, (11/10/07).

[54] "Summary Health Statistics for U.S. Children: National Health Interview Survey, 2004" Feburary 2006, U.S. Department of Health an dHuman Services, Centers for Disease Control and Prevention, National Center for Health Statistics, <http://www.cdc.gov/nchs/data/series/sr_10/sr10_227.pdf>, (11/10/07).

[55] Hitti, Miranda, September 1, 2005. "New Numbers on ADHD in U.S. Kids CDC: More than 4.4 Million U.S. Youngsters Diagnosed With ADHD," <http://www.webmd.com/add-adhd/news/20050901/new-numbers-on-adhd-in-us-kids>, (12/21/2007).

[56] Kane, Anthony, M.D., "ADHD and Food Allergies," December 24, 2004, <http://searchwarp.com/swa4309.htm>, (11/10/07).

[57] Jacobson, Michael, "ADHD & Diet: How Food Affects Mood," Issue 101, July/August 2000, <http://www.mothering.com/articles/growing_child/education/adhd.html>, (11/10/07).

[58] Jacobson, Michael, "ADHD & Diet: How Food Affects Mood," Issue 101, July/August 2000, <http://www.mothering.com/articles/growing_child/education/adhd.html>, (11/10/07).

[59] Jacobson, Michael F., Ph.D., and Schardt, David, M.S., "Diet, ADHD and Behavior," Center for Science in the Public Interest 1999, <http://www.cspinet.org/new/adhd_resch_bk02.pdf>, (11/10/07).

[60] Thurnell-Read, Jane, "Allergy Equals Addiction," <http://www.shareware123.com/articles/part9/allergy_equals_addiction.htm>, (11/10/07).

[61] Immuno Laboratories, Inc., "A simple blood test can help manage ADHD, middle ear infections and other childhood disorders," <http://www.betterhealthusa.com/public/165.cfm>, (11/10/07).

[62] Dr. Braly's Allergy Relief, the Natural Way, "IgG ELISA Delayed Food Allergy Testing...", <http://www.drbralyallergyrelief.com/igg.html>, (12/21/2007).

[63] Jacobson, Michael, "ADHD & Diet: How Food Affects Mood," Issue 101, July/August 2000, <http://www.mothering.com/articles/growing_child/education/adhd.html>, (11/10/07).

[64] "Asthma Statistics," American Academy of Allergy Asthma & Immunology, <http://www.aaaai.org/media/resources/media_kit/asthma_statistics.stm>, (11/10/07).

[65] "Tips to Remember: Food allergy," American Academy of Allergy Asthma & Immunology, <http://www.aaaai.org/patients/publicedmat/tips/foodallergy.stm>, (11/10/07).

[66] Dr. Greene, "Food Allergies and Asthma," July 15, 2003, <http://www.drgreene.com/21_1630.html>, (11/10/07).

[67] "Food Allergy and Lung Disease," <http://www.nutramed.com/asthma/foodallergy.htm>, (11/10/07).

[68] Dr. Braly's Allergy Relief, the Natural Way, "IgG ELISA Delayed Food Allergy Testing...", <http://www.drbralyallergyrelief.com/igg.html>, (12/21/2007).

[69] ALCAT Food & Chemical Sensitivity Test , "Asthma, Hay Fever & Sinusitis," <http://www.alcat.info/conditions/asthma.htm>, (11/12/07).

[70] "IgE-Mediated food allergy diagnosis: Current status and new perspectives," Molecular Nutrition & Food Research, Volume 51, Issue 1 , Pages 135 - 147, 31 July 2006; Revised: 4 August 2006, <http://www3.interscience.wiley.com/cgi-bin/abstract/114032672/ABSTRACT>, (11/12/07).

[71] "Food Allergy Around World," Food Allergy & Anaphylaxis Alliance, <http://www.foodallergyalliance.org/foo.html>, (11/12/07).

[72] "Food Allergy Around World," Food Allergy & Anaphylaxis Alliance, <http://www.foodallergyalliance.org/foo.html>, (11/12/07).

[73] Wang NR, Li HQ, "Prognoses of food allergy in infancy," Department of Child Health Care, Children's Hospital Affiliated to Chongqing Medical University, Chongqing 400014, China, October 2005, <http://www.ncbi.nlm.nih.gov/sites/entrez?Db=pubmed&Cmd=Show Detail-View&TermToSearch=16255859&ordinalpos=2&itool=EntrezSystem2.PEntrez.Pubmed.Pubmed_ResultsPanel.Pubmed_RVDocSum>, (11/12/07).

[74] Hadley, Caroline, "Food allergies on the rise? Determining the prevalence of food allergies, and how quickly it is increasing is the first step in tackling the problem," November 2006, EMBO reports, <http://www.pubmedcentral.nih.gov/articlerender.fcgi?artid=167977 5>, (11/12/07).

[75] Squires, Sally, "Allergies Can Drive You Nuts," May 16, 2006, Washington Post.Com, <http://www.google.com/search?hl=en&q=china+and+peanut+allergy >, (11/12/07).

[76] Li, Xiu-Min, M.D. and Sampson, Hugh, M.D., "Theapeutic Effect of Chinese Herbal Medicine on Food Allergy", Mount Sinai School of Medicine, September 2006, <http://www.faiusa.org/section_home.cfm?section_id=7>, (11/12/07).

[77] Allergologie-Pneumologie, Hôpital des Enfants, Toulouse Cedex, France, "Prevalence and main characteristics of schoolchildren diagnosed with food allergies in France," February 2005, <http://www.ncbi.nlm.nih.gov/sites/entrez>, (11/12/07).

[78] Lukassowitz, Dr. Irene, "Allergies in Germany," 15/8/2006, BfR Federal Institute for Risk Assessment, <http://www.bfr.bund.de/cd/8291>, (11/12/07).

[79] Kumar, Dr. Latha, "All About Food Allergies," IndoIndians.com, <http://www.indoindians.com/health/food.htm>, (11/12/07).

[80] Gangal, S.V., Malik, B.K., "Food allergy: How much of a problem really is this in India?" Council of Scientific & Industrial Research, New Delhi, INDE, 2007, <http://cat.inist.fr/?aModele=afficheN&cpsidt=15008797>, (11/12/07).

[81] Dalal I, Binson I, Reifen R, Amitai Z, Shohat T, Rahmani S, Levine A, Ballin A, Somekh E., "Food allergy is a matter of geography after all: sesame as a major cause of severe IgE-mediated food allergic reactions among infants and young children in Israel," April 2002, <http://www.ncbi.nlm.nih.gov/sites/entrez?Db=pubmed&Cmd=Show Detail-View&TermToSearch=11906370&ordinalpos=1&itool=EntrezSystem2.PEntrez.Pubmed.Pubmed_ResultsPanel.Pubmed_RVAbstractPlus>, (11/12/07).

[82] Brinn, David, "Israeli scientists crack mystery of food allergies," August 15, 2004, Health, <http://www.israel21c.org/bin/en.jsp?enDispWho=Articles%5El753&enSearchQueryID=89&enPage=BlankPage&enDisplay=view&enDispWhat=object&enVersion=0&enZone=Health&>, (11/12/07).

[83] Siegel, Judy, "Study shows camel's milk helps children get over hump of food allergies," December, 12, 2005, <http://pqasb.pqarchiver.com/jpost/access/941828101.html?dids=941828101:941828101&FMT=ABS&FMTS=ABS:FT&date=Dec+12%2C+2005&author=JUDY+SIEGEL&pub=Jerusalem+Post&edition=&startpage=01&desc=Study+shows+camel%27s+milk+helps+children+get+over+hump+of+food+allergies>, (11/12/07).

[84] "Food Allergy Around World," Food Allergy & Anaphylaxis Alliance, <http://www.foodallergyalliance.org/foo.html>, (11/12/07).

[85] Shoji, Mashahiro, "Food Allergy and Legislation in Japan: Overview," Morinaga Institute of Biological Science, Inc., 11/28/2006, <http://www.hc-sc.gc.ca/fn-an/securit/allerg/workshop-atelier/masahiro_shoji_abstract_e.html>, (11/12/07).

[86] "Food Allergy Around World," Food Allergy & Anaphylaxis Alliance, <http://www.foodallergyalliance.org/foo.html>, (11/12/07).

[87] "Food Allergy Around World," Food Allergy & Anaphylaxis Alliance, <http://www.foodallergyalliance.org/foo.html>, (11/12/07).

[88] Eriksson, N. E.; Möller, C.; Werner, S.; Magnusson, J.; Bengtsson, U.; and Zolubas, M., "Self-reported food hypersensitivity in Sweden, Denmark, Estonia, Lithuania and Russia." J Invest Allergol Clin Immunol 2004; Vol. 14(1): 70-79, <http://www.jiaci.org/issues/vol14issue01-70-79.htm?jiaci=1&search=5a4bc163286542d97b61847b7898fc49>, (11/12/07).

[89] Motala, Dr Cassiem, Allergy Society of South Africa, <http://www.allergysa.org/food.htm>, (11/12/07).

[90] Immuno-allergy Laboratory, La Paz Children's Hospital, Madrid, Spain, "Frequency of food allergy in a pediatric population from Spain," February 1995, <http://www.ncbi.nlm.nih.gov/sites/entrez>, (11/12/07).

[91] "Food Allergy Around World," Food Allergy & Anaphylaxis Alliance, <http://www.foodallergyalliance.org/foo.html>, (11/12/07).

[92] "Food Allergy & Anaphylaxis Network - Docket No. 2004N-051 6 (2005 FSS)- Pu@ c Comment," <http://www.fda.gov/ohrms/DOCKETS/dockets/04n0516/04n-0516-c000001-01-vol1.pdf>, (11/7/07).

[93] "Food Allergy Around World," Food Allergy & Anaphylaxis Alliance, <http://www.foodallergyalliance.org/foo.html>, (11/12/07).

[94] "EuroPrevall aims to improve the quality of life of food allergy sufferers," <http://www.europrevall.org/>, (11/12/07).

[95] Mills, E. N. C.; Mackie, A. R.; Burney, P.; Beyer, K.; Frewer L.; Madsen, C.; Botjes, E.; Crevel, R. W. R.; van Ree, R. (2007) The prevalence, cost and basis of food allergy across Europe Allergy 62 (7), 717–722, doi:10.1111/j.1398-9995.2007.01425.x, <http://www.blackwell-synergy.com/doi/abs/10.1111/j.1398-9995.2007.01425.x?prevSearch=allfield%3A%28ghana+food+allergie s%29>, (11/12/07).

[96] The American Heritage® Dictionary of the English Language, Fourth Edition copyright ©2000 by Houghton Mifflin Company. Updated in 2003. Published by Houghton Mifflin Company, <http://www.thefreedictionary.com/anaphylactic+shock>, (12/26/2007).

[97] Barry, Joseph, M.D., "What are Food Allergies?" <http://internalmedicine.preventive-med.com/FoodAllergy.html>, (11/12/07).

[98] Food Allergy Initiative, Food Allergen Labeling & Consumer Protection Act becomes Law:
Millions of Americans Will Be Able to Easily Identify Safe and Unsafe Foods," <http://www.foodallergyinitiative.org/press_release_20040803.html>, (11/12/07).

[99] Children's Hospital of Wisconson, <http://www.chw.org/display/PPF/DocID/21929/Nav/1/router.asp>, (12/28/2007).

[100] The Food Allergy & Anaphylaxis Network, <http://www.foodallergy.org/allergens/milk.html>, (11/13/07).

[101] "Allergies, Intolerances, Food," <http://babyandkidallergies.com/dairyingredients.php>, (11/13/07).

[102] "Milk Allergy," Food Allergy Initiative, <http://www.foodallergyinitiative.org/section_home.cfm?section_id=3&sub_section_id=3>, (11/13/07).

[103] The Food Allergy & Anaphylaxis Network, <http://www.foodallergy.org/allergens/egg.html>, (11/13/07).

[104] "Egg Allergy Diet," KidsHealth, October 2003, <http://www.kidshealth.org/parent/nutrition_fit/nutrition/egg_allergy_diet.html>, (11/13/07).

[105] Pitman, Simon, "Clarins comes under fire over peanut ingredient," 11/1/2006,

<http://www.cosmeticsdesign.com/news/ng.asp?id=71743>, (11/12/07).

106 Rufle, Samantha, "Peanut Allergy: Overview," January 23, 2007, Suite101.com, <http://allergies.suite101.com/article.cfm/peanut_allergy_overview>, (11/13/07).

107 "Nut and Peanut Allergy Diet," Reviewed by: William J. Geimeier, MD, KidsHealth, September 2003, <http://www.kidshealth.org/parent/nutrition_fit/nutrition/nut_peanut_allergy_diet.html>, (11/13/07).

108 "Peanut Allergy," Food Allergy Initiative, <http://www.foodallergyinitiative.org/section_home.cfm?section_id=3&sub_section_id=1>, (11/13/07).

109 "Nut and Peanut Allergy Diet," Reviewed by: William J. Geimeier, MD, KidsHealth, September 2003, <http://www.kidshealth.org/parent/nutrition_fit/nutrition/nut_peanut_allergy_diet.html>, (11/13/07).

110 The Food Allergy & Anaphylaxis Network, <http://www.foodallergy.org/allergens/treenut.html>, (11/13/07).

111 "Tree Nut Allergy" Food Allergy Initiative, <http://www.foodallergyinitiative.org/section_home.cfm?section_id=3&sub_section_id=6>, (11/13/07).

112 Soy Allergy, 11/12/07, <http://www.allergicchild.com/soy_allergies.htm>, (11/12/07).

113 Allergies, Intolerances, Food, <http://www.babyandkidallergies.com/soyingredients.php>, (11/13/07).

114 "Soy Allergy," Food Allergy Initiative, <http://www.foodallergyinitiative.org/section_home.cfm?section_id=3&sub_section_id=7, (11/13/07)>.

[115] FAAN, "Tips for Managing a Wheat Allergy,"
<http://www.foodallergy.org/allergens/wheat.html>, (12/6/07).

[116] FAAN, "Tips for Managing a Wheat Allergy,"
<http://www.foodallergy.org/allergens/wheat.html>, (12/6/07).

[117] National Digestive Diseases Information Clearinghouse, "Celiac Disease,"
August 2007, <http://digestive.niddk.nih.gov/ddiseases/pubs/celiac/>,
(11/12/07).

[118] National Digestive Diseases Information Clearinghouse, "Celiac Disease,"
August 2007, <http://digestive.niddk.nih.gov/ddiseases/pubs/celiac/>,
(11/12/07).

[119] The University of Chicago Celiac Disease Center, "Living with Celiac Disease," <http://www.celiacdisease.net/gluten-free-diet>, (11/12/07).

[120] "Wheat Allergy," Food Allergy Initiative,
<http://www.foodallergyinitiative.org/section_home.cfm?section_id=3
&sub_section_id=5>, (11/13/07).

[121] "Tips for Managing a Fish and/or Shellfish Allergy,"
<http://www.foodallergy.org/allergens/fish.html>, (11/12/07).

[122] "Seafood Allergy,"
2005,<http://www.aafa.org/display.cfm?id=9&sub=20&cont=518>,
(11/12/07).

[123] Australian Museum Fish Site, <http://www.amonline.net.au/fishes/>,
(12/28/2007).

[124] "Fish Allergy," Food Allergy Initiative,
<http://www.foodallergyinitiative.org/section_home.cfm?section_id=3
&sub_section_id=8>, (11/13/07).

[125] "Shellfish Allergy," Food Allergy Initiative,
<http://www.foodallergyinitiative.org/section_home.cfm?section_id=3
&sub_section_id=4>, (11/13/07).

[126] "Shellfish & Fish Allergy," AllergicChild.com, 11/12/07, <http://www.allergicchild.com/shellfish_allergy.htm>, (11/13/07).

[127] "TITLE 21--FOOD AND DRUGS, CHAPTER I--FOOD AND DRUG ADMINISTRATION, DEPARTMENT OF HEALTH AND HUMAN SERVICES, FOOD LABELING, Sec. 101.22 Foods; labeling of spices, flavorings, colorings and chemical preservatives," <http://www.cfsan.fda.gov/~lrd/CF101-22.HTML>, (11/14/07).

[128] "TITLE 21--FOOD AND DRUGS, CHAPTER I--FOOD AND DRUG ADMINISTRATION, DEPARTMENT OF HEALTH AND HUMAN SERVICES, FOOD LABELING, Sec. 101.22 Foods; labeling of spices, flavorings, colorings and chemical preservatives," <http://www.cfsan.fda.gov/~lrd/CF101-22.HTML>, (11/14/07).

[129] Schlosser, Eric, "Fast Food Nation II," 1/23/03, <http://www.thetruthseeker.co.uk/article.asp?ID=130>, (11/14/07).

[130] "Food Color Facts," U. S. Food and Drug Administration FDA/IFIC* Brochure: January 1993, <http://www.cfsan.fda.gov/~lrd/colorfac.html>, (11/14/07).

[131] "TITLE 21--FOOD AND DRUGS, CHAPTER I--FOOD AND DRUG ADMINISTRATION, DEPARTMENT OF HEALTH AND HUMAN SERVICES, PART 70--COLOR ADDITIVES," <http://frwebgate2.access.gpo.gov/cgi-bin/waisgate.cgi?WAISdocID=049794503514+8+0+0&WAISaction=retrieve>, (11/14/07).

[132] "TITLE 21--FOOD AND DRUGS, CHAPTER I--FOOD AND DRUG ADMINISTRATION, DEPARTMENT OF HEALTH AND HUMAN SERVICES, PART 70--COLOR ADDITIVES," <http://frwebgate2.access.gpo.gov/cgi-bin/waisgate.cgi?WAISdocID=049794503514+8+0+0&WAISaction=retrieve>, (11/14/07).

[133] Quinn, Jeannette, "Natural colors in dairy foods: maintaining a natural ingredient statement and providing consumer-appealing color - Ingredient Technology Focus," Dairy Foods, April, 2003,

<http://findarticles.com/p/articles/mi_m3301/is_4_104/ai_100573011>
, (11/14/07).

134 "TITLE 21--FOOD AND DRUGS, CHAPTER I--FOOD AND DRUG
ADMINISTRATION, DEPARTMENT OF HEALTH AND HUMAN
SERVICES, PART 70--COLOR ADDITIVES,"
<http://frwebgate2.access.gpo.gov/cgi-
bin/waisgate.cgi?WAISdocID=049794503514+8+0+0&WAISaction=r
etrieve>, (11/14/07).

135 "TITLE 21--FOOD AND DRUGS, CHAPTER I--FOOD AND DRUG
ADMINISTRATION, DEPARTMENT OF HEALTH AND HUMAN
SERVICES, FOOD LABELING, Sec. 101.22 Foods; labeling of
spices, flavorings, colorings and chemical preservatives,"
<http://www.cfsan.fda.gov/~lrd/CF101-22.HTML>, (11/14/07).

136 Raloff, Janet, "The mango that thought it was poison ivy," Food for
Thought by Science News and Science Services,
<http://www.sciencenews.org/pages/sn_arc98/8_8_98/food.htm>,
(11/14/07).

137 Raloff, Janet, "The mango that thought it was poison ivy," Food for
Thought by Science News and Science Services,
<http://www.sciencenews.org/pages/sn_arc98/8_8_98/food.htm>,
(11/14/07).

138 Raloff, Janet, "The mango that thought it was poison ivy," Food for
Thought by Science News and Science Services,
<http://www.sciencenews.org/pages/sn_arc98/8_8_98/food.htm>,
(11/14/07).

139 "Tree Nuts – One of the nine most common food allergens," Canadian Food
Inspection Agency developed in consultation with Allergy/Asthma
Information Association, Anaphylaxis Canada,
<http://www.inspection.gc.ca/english/fssa/labeti/allerg/nutnoie.shtml
>, (11/14/07).

140 Vieths, S.; Scheurer, S.; Ballmer-Weber, B., "Current understanding of
cross-reactivity of food allergens and pollen," Paul-Ehrlich-Institut,
Department of Allergology, Paul-Ehrlich-Str. 51-59, D-63225 Lan-
gen, Germany. Viest@pei.de, May 2002,

<http://www.ncbi.nlm.nih.gov/sites/entrez?Db=pubmed&Cmd=Show
Detail-
View&TermToSearch=12023194&ordinalpos=9&itool=EntrezSys-
tem2.PEntrez.Pubmed.Pubmed_ResultsPanel.Pubmed_RVDocSum>,
(11/14/07).

141 "Food Allergy – An Overview," U.S. DEPARTMENT OF HEALTH AND
HUMAN SERVICES, National Institutes of Health, National Institute of Allergy and Infectious Diseases, July 2007,
<http://www.niaid.nih.gov/publications/pdf/foodallergy.pdf>,
(11/14/07).

142 Ellis-Christensen, Tricia, "What are the Effects of an Iodine Allergy?"
WiseGEEK, <http://www.wisegeek.com/what-are-the-effects-of-an-
iodine-allergy.htm>, (11/14/07).

143 "The Probiotic Leader: Functions of Probiotic Species," Reprinted with
permission of Klaire Labs, a division of ProThera, Inc. Reno, NV,
http://www.klaire.com/probioticleader3.htm, (3/26/2008).

144 "Probiotics Help Local Kids with Food Allergies," The Boston Parents Paper, December 2007, <http://boston.parenthood.com/?segid=138>,
(12/30/07).

145 Food Allergy & Anaphylaxis Network - Docket No. 2004N-051 6 (2005
FSS) - Public Comment,
<http://www.fda.gov/ohrms/DOCKETS/dockets/04n0516/04n-0516-
c000001-01-vol1.pdf>, (2/26/08).

146 "Allergy Alert," DKLT Kids, <http://www.dltk-
kids.com/recipes/allergyalert.html>, (11/14/07).

147 "Allergy Alert," DKLT Kids, <http://www.dltk-
kids.com/recipes/allergyalert.html>, (11/14/07).

148 Parentingscience.com, "The dark side of preschool: Peers, social skills, and
stress," <http://www.parentingscience.com/preschool-stress.html>,
(11/15/07).

[149] Parentingscience.com, "The dark side of preschool: Peers, social skills, and stress," <http://www.parentingscience.com/preschool-stress.html>, (11/15/07).

[150] Lelchuk, Ilene, "California UC study examines preschool benefits by third grade, no difference shown among students," January, 27 2006, San Francisco Chronicle, <http://www.sfgate.com/cgi-bin/article.cgi?f=/c/a/2006/01/27/BAG8AGTL0E1.DTL>, (11/15/07).

[151] Olsen, Darcy Ann, "Preschool in the Nanny State," Weekly Standard, August 9, 1999, Education and Child Policy, the CATO Institute, <http://www.cato.org/research/education/articles/nannystate.html>, (11/15/07).

[152] "Professors Find Preschool Benefits Grossly Exaggerated: Errors in Rand's cost-benefit analysis caused sever over-estimation of preschool benefits," The Reason Foundation, <http://www.reason.org/news/universalpreschool_053006.shtml>, (11/15/07).

[153] "Getting Your Child Ready for Kindergarten," <http://www.sde.ct.gov/sde/lib/sde/PDF/DEPS/Early/KinderBroEng.pdf>, (11/15/07).

[154] "Protecting Students with Disabilities: Frequently Asked Questions About Sectin 504 and the Education of Children with Disabilities," 3/4/05, U.S. Department of Education, <http://www.ed.gov/about/offices/list/ocr/504faq.html>, (11/15/07).

[155] Groce, Victoria, "Food Allergies in Schools: Do You Need a 504 Plan for Food Allergy?" October 5, 2007, About.com: Food Allergies, <http://foodallergies.about.com/od/adultfoodallergies/i/504planprocon.htm>, (11/14/07).

[156] "Living with Food Allergies: Section 504 Plan Outline," <http://www.foodallergyinitiative.org/section_home.cfm?section_id=4&sub_section_id=4&article_id=35>, (11/15/07).

157 "Action Plan for Anaphylaxis," ASCIA 2003, <http://www.medeserv.com.au/ascia/aer/infobulletins/posters/Anaphy laxis_plan_(child)_Au.pdf>, (11/15/07).

158 "What Can You Bring on the Airplane?", August 10, 2006, Good Morning America, <http://abcnews.go.com/GMA/story?id=2295674>, (11/15/07).

159 Plowright, Teresa, "Rules for Carry-On Luggage," About.com: Family Vacations, <http://travelwithkids.about.com/od/planetrips/qt/carry_on.htm>, (11/15/07).

160 Groce, Victoria, "Airline Allergy Policies," About.com: Food Allergies, August 17, 2007, <http://foodallergies.about.com/od/livingwithfoodallergies/a/airlinepo licies.htm>, (11/15/07).

161 "International '911' and Emergency Numbers," Santa Clara County Fire Department, <http://www.sccfd.org/travel.html>, (11/15/07).

162 "H.R. 2063: Food Allergy and Anaphylaxis Management Act of 2008," GovTrack.us, http://www.govtrack.us/congress/bill.xpd?bill=h110-2063&tab=summary, (5/24/2008).

163 Sheehan, Charles, "Scientists see spike in kids' food allergies," Chicago Tribune, 9 June 2006, <http://www.non-gm-farmers.com/news_details.asp?ID=2789>, (12/31/2007).